· HOW TO ·
LOOK & FEEL
HALF YOUR AGE

For the rest of your Life

· HOW TO ·
LOOK & FEEL
HALF YOUR AGE

For the rest of your Life

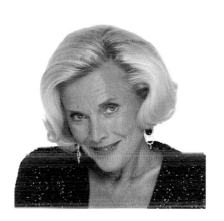

Virgin

With exclusive photography by
John Rogers

First published in 1997 by Virgin Books,
an imprint of Virgin Publishing Ltd
332 Ladbroke Grove, London W10 5AH

A catalogue record for this book is available from the British Library

ISBN:1 85227 607 X
Colour separations by :Pendry Litho Hove England
Printed and bound in Great Britain by
Butler & Tanner Ltd, Frome and London

Text by Honor Blackman with Jane O'Gorman
All special photography by John Rogers
Designed by Haldane Mason
For Virgin Publishing: Carolyn Price

CONTENTS

CLOTHES FOR THE FASHION SHOOT COURTESY OF **MaxMara**

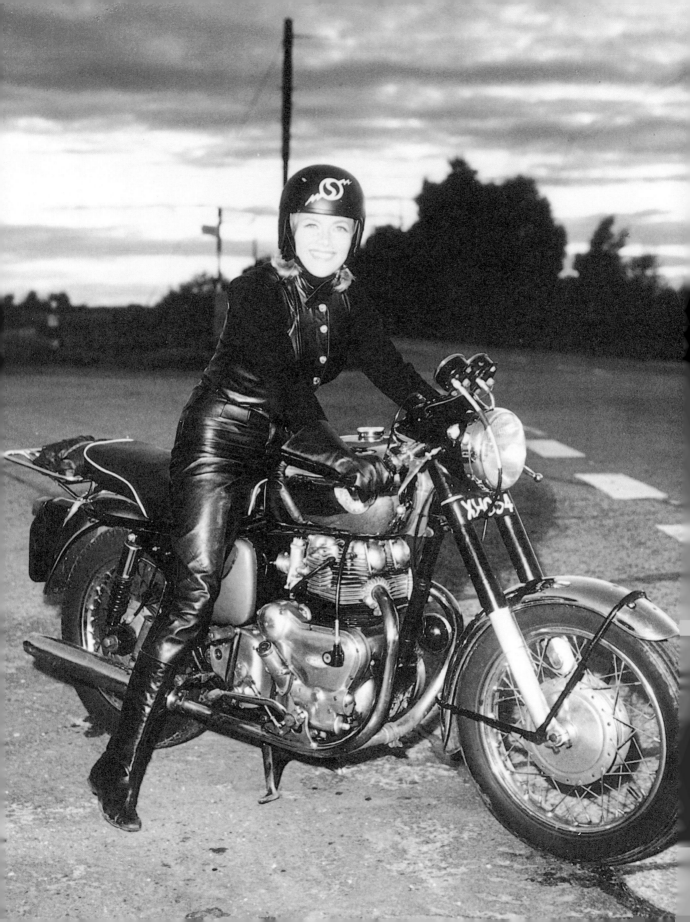

Foreword

As women we are constantly being pulled in different directions, as mothers, wives, friends and employees and it seems that there is always someone else who requires our time and attention. I've written this book as a reminder to every woman who reads it that although the needs of others are important, **you** are important too.

My life is a rich mixture of work, social life and family commitments but I make sure that it in no way prevents me from eating sensibly, exercizing regularly and getting enough sleep. I'm frequently asked how I seem to be so full of life. Well, there is no secret, no magic potions I could recommend you use. I look healthy because I am. I have a lot of energy because my diet is sensible but not rigid, my exercise routine is regular but not killing and my appetite for life as healthy as it ever was. Being fit doesn't mean I'm a fitness fanatic; people never seem to equate being fit and healthy with having fun, but the whole point of exercise is to be in such good form that you are able to approach your work with more vigour and enthusiasm and really enjoy your leisure hours.

I suggest you organize your life so that you can incorporate some of the tips I've included in this book. Make the extra effort and you will find that getting and staying fit and healthy becomes easier every day. I have always believed that I am worth spending time on - and worth making an effort for - perhaps that is my secret?

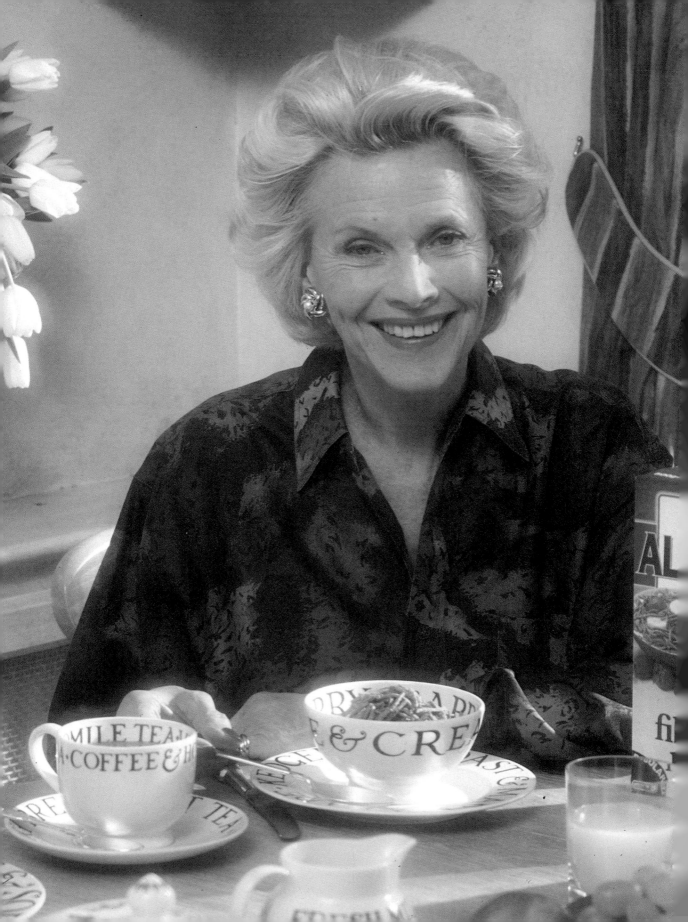

EATING WELL, FEELING BETTER

I have a great appetite for life. I actually enjoy waking up in the morning and look forward to what the day will bring. It isn't necessarily all good of course, but I think that if you are well slept, well fed and reasonably well organized then you can cope better with all eventualities. Part of my appetite for life includes my appetite for food. I love to eat. To me, food is an indulgent pleasure. Whether it's a freshly cut cheese sandwich oozing with HP Sauce (a particular favourite of mine) or a dish of delicious profiteroles stuffed with wicked double cream, I love to give my taste buds a treat especially if someone else is cooking.

I've often said that I'd rather go through the agonies of a first night than have to cook a three-course meal for six people. I'm not a natural in the kitchen, cooking doesn't fascinate me and I've had my share of disasters just like everyone else, but that doesn't in the least detract from my love of food. If a friend suggests that we go out for the evening I like nothing better than to visit a super restaurant and sample the best the chef has to offer. To me, food equates socializing, good health and fun. One of my great weaknesses is for old-fashioned sticky puddings. In The *Upper Hand* company I'm famous for heading the queue in the Carlton canteen when syrup sponge is on the menu. When we made the first episode of *The Upper Hand* our producer, Christopher Walker, took it to Los Angeles to run it for Columbia studios, who had originated the show in the States under the title *Who's The Boss?*

CONTENTS

Since Columbia Studios were familiar with my work it was commented upon that I looked in very good nick for a lady of my age (I hate that comment — you notice that people so rarely say that sort of thing about men!). Christopher, having rather a wicked sense of humour, said, 'Oh yes, and you should see her in the canteen, she eats everything. Her favourite is spotted dick.' This dish is completely unfamiliar to the Americans and you can imagine their reaction.

Some weeks later, back in the British studio, Christopher whispered to me that I'd get a surprise at lunchtime — and what was on the menu? Spotted dick, for the first time. Now jam roly poly, syrup sponge or spotted dick are always on the menu when Carlton know we're having our studio day.

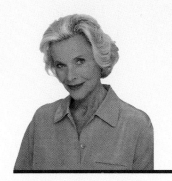

'Everything I buy is fresh, fresh, fresh. There is no other way to stay fit.'

I find that I can indulge myself with naughty puddings once in a while because I strike a balance with all the other foods I eat the rest of the time. Luckily we're only at the studio for one day a week when making *The Upper Hand*, so the puddings aren't ruinous. The rest of the time I thrive on fresh vegetables (organic ones, if I can get them — they taste better), a huge variety of fish and just a little meat.

And make no mistake, even when I'm alone, which is quite often, I cook fresh vegetables and fresh everything else too. I think I've eaten three chill-cook meals in my life and two of those were when I was out with friends.

I always try to follow the advice of top chefs and buy the best produce I can afford as I'd rather have a little bit of something really good than a plateful of mediocrity. You won't find me swanning around the food halls of Harrods or Fortnum & Mason buying the most expensive food I can find. I pride myself on being a very discerning and canny shopper. I shop in street markets, locally run businesses and supermarkets alike — anywhere that the best-quality food is on sale.

I always try to eat three good meals a day, although if you've worked for years in the theatre as I have, eating late is a habit that dies hard and of course it is terribly bad for the digestive system. Angela Lansbury once told me that she never eats anything after 7pm at night and that's a habit I'd like to get into, although in reality I don't imagine I ever shall. Instead I discipline myself to eat sensibly and allow myself to be unwise only when I'm out with friends. I hate to be one of those people who when presented with some delicious pudding says, 'Oh no, I daren't.' Your hosts have gone to a huge amount of trouble preparing it for you, the very least they deserve is the courtesy of you eating it. Besides which, I love anything homemade and gooey. One friend of mine says 'It's all right, there IS a pudding' as I walk into her house for a meal because she knows that I love desserts.

My trick is that I treat myself only when I feel I deserve it and the plan seems to work. With the help of plenty of exercise I've been about the same weight for as long as I can remember. I'm 5ft 5½in tall and weigh 8st 12lb. If I look good it's because I eat and drink sensibly and have good genes – and before you say 'There you are, it's all in the genes', I have one sister who is skinnier than I and one who both of us would fit into. I also had an aunt who had to go through the door sideways. So you see, the genes do need assistance.

WHIPPING UP A TREAT

Because I'm not a natural in the kitchen, when I'm at home with my family I like to eat simply and well. I try to avoid over-processed foods and will always buy fresh fruit and vegetables whenever I can. I have a great respect for food and eat as much to keep healthy as to satisfy my appetite. I'm lucky in that I can eat almost anything. I don't suffer from food allergies and I really look forward to my next meal.

I don't like preparing fiddly dishes or fussy sauces that take hours to put together. I've been to so many dinner parties over the years where the hostess has tried desperately to do something complicated and ultimately ends up by putting a meal on the table which is overambitious and lukewarm.

On the rare occasions when I entertain I much prefer to steam a whole fish or concoct something like a huge casserole which allows me to feed my guests AND join in the conversation. I hate being left out and believe that eating with family and friends should be a fun, pleasurable, shared experience and not something to be slaved over.

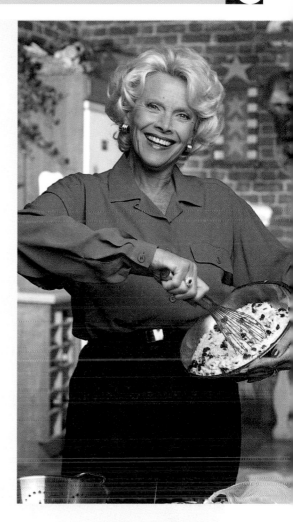

I love to eat spotted dick but it's not often that you'll actually see me cooking it!

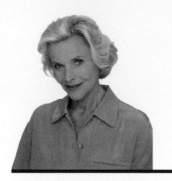

'Keeping in shape is vital to me. If we are what we eat then I am a testimony to that.'

Fans of *The Upper Hand* will notice that my character, Laura West, is never seen with a pinny tied around her middle whipping up a little something in the kitchen. She's more likely to be whipping up a little something in the bedroom. Maybe that's why I enjoy playing her so much.

I like to keep in shape because I can't bear the feel of a spare tyre developing and they develop very quickly, especially after a certain age! It isn't just vanity. It makes me feel like a pudding and not a bit 'vibrant' (that's my dear Patrick Macnee's favourite word). So eating correctly and exercising are very important to me.

In any case, I have to get up on stage in front of hundreds of people a night or be seen by millions when I'm on television and I would hate it for anyone to say 'Goodness, hasn't she put weight on round her stomach' or a similar charming remark.

Of course this applies to the characters I am at present playing. Some actors are employed because of their rotundity, but which came first, the chicken or the egg? I doubt if many of them would claim that they had developed their girth specifically to get work. It never ceases to amaze me that a man can have one of those ghastly big stomachs hanging over his belt and people rarely say 'Heavens, you look gross.' A beer belly is treated almost with affection. I can't think why, as they are hideous. However, if a woman puts on weight then everyone comments on it.

GET THE BALANCE RIGHT

I think that I have a healthy approach to eating. It's not faddy, it's not trendy and doesn't involve expensive meal replacement milk shakes or packet foods. I've never dieted in my life — on the contrary, there have been times when I've often wished that I could actually put weight on, especially around my thighs. But I don't look as I do by accident — I buy fresh, natural foods and cook them simply. If I come across some delicious fresh peas in the market then I'll pod them nightly while they are in season as an accompaniment to almost anything — I love their delicate, sweet flavour. I enjoy a rich variety of foods and I certainly don't believe in eating things that I don't like even if they are supposed to be good for me. Take bean sprouts, for instance – I can't stand them. You are as likely to find me eating bean sprouts as wasting my time whisking up a fiddly soufflé.

I buy free range foods when I can. I don't deny myself the odd chocolate or the occasional helping of syrup sponge because I enjoy them. Often friends coming to dinner bring gorgeous boxes of chocolates and I make sure to remember to hand them around that night as trying to ration myself during the following week is something of a strain. But I do deliberately provide treats for myself sometimes. For example, if I have lines to learn or fan mail to get through I provide myself with something delicious to look forward to when the job is done. We don't grow up, it's just a 'sweetie' for the good child.

You will know that certain foods are bad for you from both the health and weight point of view, so if you are aware that you are incapable of indulging in them in moderation, just don't touch them at all.

I think the lives of too many women have been made miserable by yo-yo dieting and food trends in recent years. The endless cycle of dieting, bingeing and guilt has made a lot of women very unhappy.

I can certainly sympathize with women who have tried every fashionable diet under the sun and still find that they are a size 18 after years of meticulous calorie counting. But dieting and then lapsing are so bad for you. Organize yourself into eating sensibly – permanently. There is so much that tastes good that you don't have to deprive yourself, for heaven's sake. What has always worked for me in keeping my weight steady is a healthy eating plan coupled with plenty of activity. Activities like walking the dog, cleaning the windows and doing the gardening count too.

I remember a famous actress once said, 'Women who do all of their own housework don't need to go to the gym.' Well, I do both.

If you are actively trying to lose weight then remember that you are an individual and that everybody's metabolism is unique. You may find that by re-educating yourself into eating a balanced

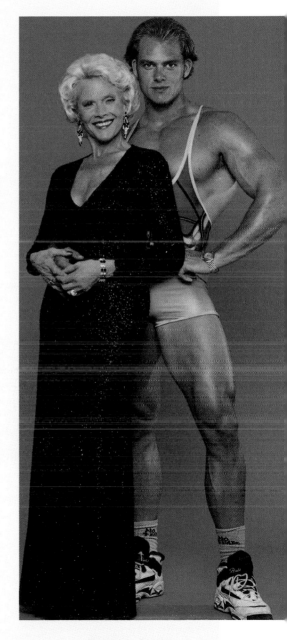

Hunter, my favourite Gladiator – a man who hasn't let himself go!

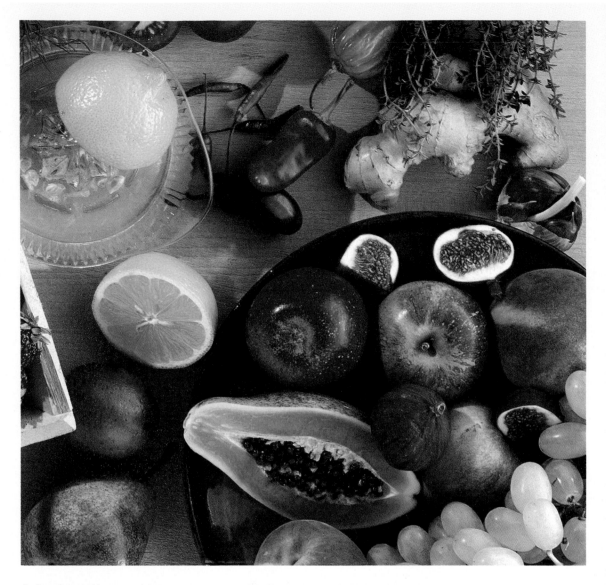

Fruit and vegetables
bursting with essential
vitamins are my first,
second and third choice.

diet and taking more exercise you lose a lot of weight in the first
month and then nothing for the next couple of weeks.

- *Don't give up*
- *Set a realistic target weight*
- *Aim to lose about a pound a week*
- *Allow yourself a treat every now and then*
- *Think positively.*

Once you reach your goal you'll feel really good about
yourself, have bags more energy and have the perfect excuse
to treat yourself to that sexy new outfit – and then you'll have

to keep up your new regime so that the outfit continues to fit.

Basically, to lose weight our bodies need to burn up more energy than they take in. This means less fattening foods and drinks and more physical activity. But remember, it's just as important to avoid being underweight as overweight. Being underweight can lead to osteoporosis (thinning of the bones), while obesity increases the risk of diabetes and heart disease.

Each day, ensure that your intake is balanced by eating a variety of foods from the following main food groups:

- *Fruit and vegetables*
- *Bread, other cereals and potatoes*
- *Milk and dairy products*
- *Meat, fish and other proteins (like nuts and pulses).*

Roughly speaking, one third of your daily intake should be fruit and vegetables, one third starch (bread, etc.) and one third meat and dairy products. It's not the bread or potatoes that will make you fat – they are wonderful fibre providers – it's the butter or cheese you put on them that does the damage.

VITAMINS, NATURALLY

I believe that it's always preferable, where possible, to get vitamins from natural food sources:

- *Vitamin A: This can be found in dairy products, fish, liver, carrots, eggs, margarine and dark leafy vegetables like broccoli. It is needed for healthy eyes, teeth, lungs and skin, and for fighting infection. Never take extra Vitamin A if you are pregnant or planning to conceive.*
- *Vitamin B group: There are a large number of vitamins in the B group. B1 and B2 are found in brewer's yeast, cereals and meat, B3 in liver, tuna and peanuts, B5 and B6 in liver, whole grains and egg yolks, B12 in shellfish, Marmite and meat. These are needed for many purposes, including promoting a healthy nervous system, healthy hair and red blood-cell formation.*
- *Beta-carotene: This turns into vitamin A when you eat it. It is found mainly in yellow and orange fruits and vegetables such as apricots, peaches, carrots and sweet potatoes. It may offer protection against heart disease and cancers of the breast, lung and bladder.*
- *Vitamin C: Most citrus fruits and vegetables including tomatoes and*

TOP TIPS

- Ideally we should eat at least five different varieties of fruit and vegetable a day. I know it's difficult in a busy life, but do try.
- I find that it's best to fill up with starchy foods like pasta, rice and bread when I get really hungry rather than reaching for the biscuit tin and instantly regretting it.
- I try not to make meat the main part of any meal. I find that if I prepare delicious vegetables meat becomes a secondary consideration.
- Eating a little and often is always the best way to balance the body's sugar levels. Skipping meals makes the body think that you are starving and the result is lethargy as the body slows down and stores energy.
- I avoid white flour and white sugar and aim to steam, poach or grill foods rather than frying them as much as possible.
- The best way to enjoy any fresh vegetables, in fact, is to cut them up into chunks and eat them raw. That way you can be sure of getting the very best of the food without cooking the life out of it.
- Healthy food doesn't have to be tasteless, either, now that there are so many fresh herbs on sale. I like to buy those little pots of planted herbs from the supermarket and keep them on my kitchen window sill. Or, of course, if you have a garden you can grow them. When I need fresh herbs for a dish I can simply pick them myself.
- If you get the balance of your diet right, you won't need to buy expensive vitamin supplements.

green peppers contain Vitamin C. It is good for boosting the immune system, fighting infection, promoting healthy bones and teeth and helping in the absorption of iron.

- *Vitamin D: Found in margarines, oily fish, liver and eggs, Vitamin D is also added to many fortified breakfast cereals. It is formed in the skin by direct sunlight. It is needed for proper bone formation and works in conjunction with calcium.*
- *Vitamin E: Found in vegetable oils (peanut, soya, corn), egg yolks, leafy vegetables such as brussels sprouts, cereals, sprouted seeds and beans (like alfalfa and mung beans), Vitamin E acts as an antioxidant, protects against heart disease and helps the body to create and maintain red blood cells.*
- *Vitamin K: This is found in green leafy vegetables and liver. It aids blood clotting, maintains bones and is present in the intestine.*

In addition calcium is needed for good teeth and bones and is found in dried fruit, dairy produce, bread and flour. Iron is also vital for healthy muscles and blood and is found in egg yolks, liver and chocolate!

MY SHOPPING TIPS

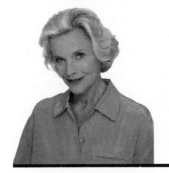

'Stop yourself impulse-buying junk foods by making a list.'

When you go shopping, do as I do and take a real interest in what you buy. Many packaged foods now have lists of the calories and nutrients contained therein as well as the E numbers to which some people may have an allergic reaction, so always check before you choose and look out for low-calorie versions of your favourite cheeses, yoghurts and soups. It's even possible to buy low-calorie cakes these days. (I have a friend who has recently had a heart attack and become diabetic. She therefore has to keep sugar and fats out of her diet but she still makes the most wonderful cakes by using recipes from a diabetic cookbook. Her whole attitude in the kitchen has changed.)

Always buy the freshest produce you can find and opt for whichever fruits and vegetables are seasonal as they will be the most delicious. You may be tempted to buy heaps of convenience foods but they really are very expensive, usually contain tiny portions and are often heavily seasoned. Opt instead for fresh foods which can be quickly steamed, stir-fried or grilled (broiled).

KEEP DRINKING

It is a good idea to keep the body constantly hydrated and refreshed by drinking plenty of liquids. As well as drinking at least 1.2 litres (2pt/5 cups) a day of filtered water I also enjoy fruit juices and mint tea.

I drink tea but I'm aware that like coffee it contains caffeine, so I tend to restrict my intake. If I have coffee after lunch, at bedtime I am ready to dance on the ceiling. According to the Department of Health an occasional alcoholic drink is likely to do you more good than harm, but too much alcohol may cause strokes and may make you more likely to develop high blood pressure and some cancers. On top of that, it's full of calories, too. One pint of beer, for example, contains more than three times the calories in a slice of bread.

Up until a couple of years ago I used to enjoy half a bottle of wine in the evening with my meal simply because I liked it. I cut it out for two weeks just to prove to myself that I could and found that the spare tyre that I had been developing had disappeared. It had not occurred to me that the wine had contributed to it.

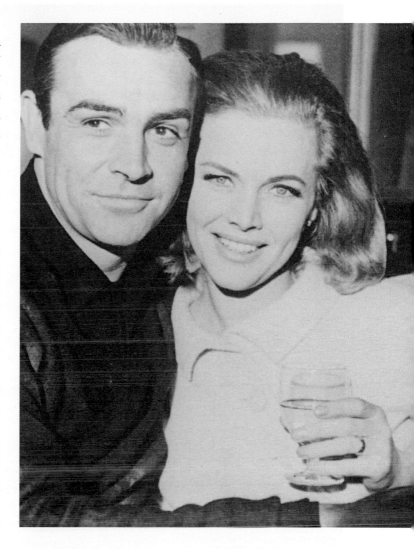

Vino Galore: Sean Connery and I during the making of *Goldfinger*. I may not have been shaken but I was definitely stirred!

These days when I go out for dinner or enjoy a meal with friends I rarely have more than a couple of glasses of wine or good champagne, which I love. If I'm at a party I may drink the occasional vodka or if I feel I need to cheer myself up I'll have a whisky. But if I was told I could never drink again I don't think it would bother me terribly. I'd be very sorry not to enjoy the taste of wine but it wouldn't be the end of the world.

It's now recommended that women should take no more than 2-3 units of alcohol a day. Units are worked out as:

* *One single measure of spirits*
* *One small glass of sherry*

- *One single measure of aperitifs*
- *One small glass of wine*
- *A half pint of ordinary strength beer, lager or cider.*

Some women, apparently, react differently to alcohol at certain times of the month. It's possible that during ovulation (which is about two weeks before a period) and also during the two or three days immediately preceding a period, the effects of alcohol are felt more quickly than at other times. It's also possible that you'll find that alcohol affects you faster once you have passed the menopause. It may be unfair, but it does seem that women's bodies are more sensitive to alcohol than those of men. I know I get terrible headaches if I exceed two glasses.

I find that a refreshing alternative to alcohol on a summer's day is to peel soft fruits and put them through the juicer to make a vitamin-C packed cocktail. Alternatively, if I fancy something

I adore fish and eat masses of it. Here I am at the fish counter of Planet Organic in London.

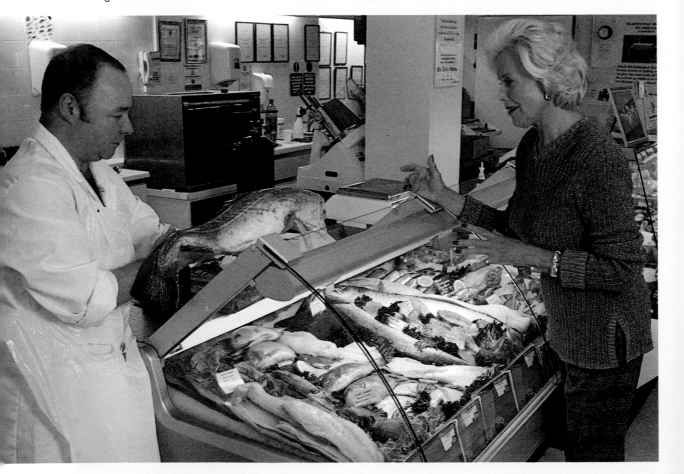

more substantial then I'll chop up a banana and add it to a large glass of skimmed milk and a few ice cubes in the blender. Whizzing it all together for a couple of seconds produces a delicious, nutritious milkshake.

One rule which I find works very well for me is never to drink anything at all with food. I don't count wine as I drink so little. I find my digestive system gets a better chance if I keep things simple and don't mix food and liquid. I always eat my food slowly and chew each mouthful properly (a rule left over from my childhood; we were taught to chew each mouthful 48 times.) Some 'bolters' die of boredom waiting for me to finish. My intake of water comes before breakfast and between meals. As I practically never suffer from indigestion it's something that I'm happy to carry on with.

MY DAY

If you want to understand how eating healthily fits into my busy life then here is a run down of a typical day in the Blackman dining room.

Breakfast

- *The first thing I do when I get up in the morning is drink 600ml (1pt/2¹/₂ cups) of purified water. I've been doing this for at least a year now and certainly feel better for it. I do leave the rehearsal room more often than others but they've become accustomed to it! I try to follow this by drinking the same amount by the afternoon. It was something a homeopath suggested I do. As our skin is made up of at least 70 per cent water, I've realized that replenishing it is vital for everyone, no matter what their age.*

- *A cup of tea follows, which is usually Indian.*

- *Next comes cereal and for me a big bowl of muesli with all sorts of nuts and fruit in it is sheer bliss. I'm also a big fan of All Bran and porridge and eat them all with semi-skimmed milk. I tend to steer clear of big fried breakfasts — frankly I find them too fatty and heavy.*

- *If I really feel like an elevenses treat then I'll have a buttery croissant or some wholemeal bread smeared with butter and a big dollop of thick marmalade. I hate margarine but I quite like the new ranges of 'pretend' butters.*

Lunch

- Lunch is vital for me because I can't go for a long time without eating. Cold chicken with salad, fresh soup and bread or something very easy like a boiled egg with soldiers are what I'll often choose.
- I always buy free range eggs although I can't say that I've ever noticed a great deal of difference in the taste.
- If I don't cheat and buy myself one of those wonderful cartons of fresh soup which are now on sale everywhere I'll occasionally have some homemade soup. It's so easy to simply sweat some vegetables with a little chopped potato and onion in a blob of butter, add some vegetable stock, cook for 20 minutes and blend the mixture until smooth then serve with a sprinkling of fresh parsley on top.
- Baked potatoes are a great favourite and are a fun food for kids too, with a choice of toppings.
- Fruit is an important part of my diet but as I'm not particularly taken with raw fruit I tend to stew or bake it. There's nothing more delicious than stewed plums or apricots with a dollop of Greek yoghurt on top or a whole apple baked with cinnamon and sultanas — and there's no need to add sugar, either, because there is plenty of natural sweetness in the fruits themselves.
- Other lunchtime desserts I enjoy include yoghurt and honey or raspberries and fromage frais.

Snack

- If I get hungry between meals I'll snack on a banana, which I always think of as being nature's perfect fast food, or some toast.
- I'm also a great fan of Ryvita (I actually like it, which surprises a lot of my friends) and I'll put almost anything on top from cheddar cheese with HP sauce to marmalade. I often use it as a substitute for bread.
- I rarely have junk food like crisps or biscuits — they contain too much fat, sugar and 'empty' calories for my liking.

Dinner

- If I'm cooking a family dinner at home we'll invariably have a big fish or a vegetarian Indian meal. My son is a coeliac (which means he has to eat a gluten-free diet) and a vegetarian so the menu is necessarily limited.
- I am always inclined to serve up at least two vegetables — which will

---

FANCY THAT

I read recently that scientists at Reading University have discovered that a little bit of what you fancy really does do you good.

Academics from ARISE – Associates for Research Into the Science of Enjoyment – say savouring the good things in life, without feeling guilty, can reduce stress and even increase resistance to disease.

Apparently they've found that the pleasure we derive from good food or an occasional glass of wine 'inoculates' the brain and reduces stress hormones. So my occasional square of chocolate or portion of syrup sponge may actually be doing me some good!

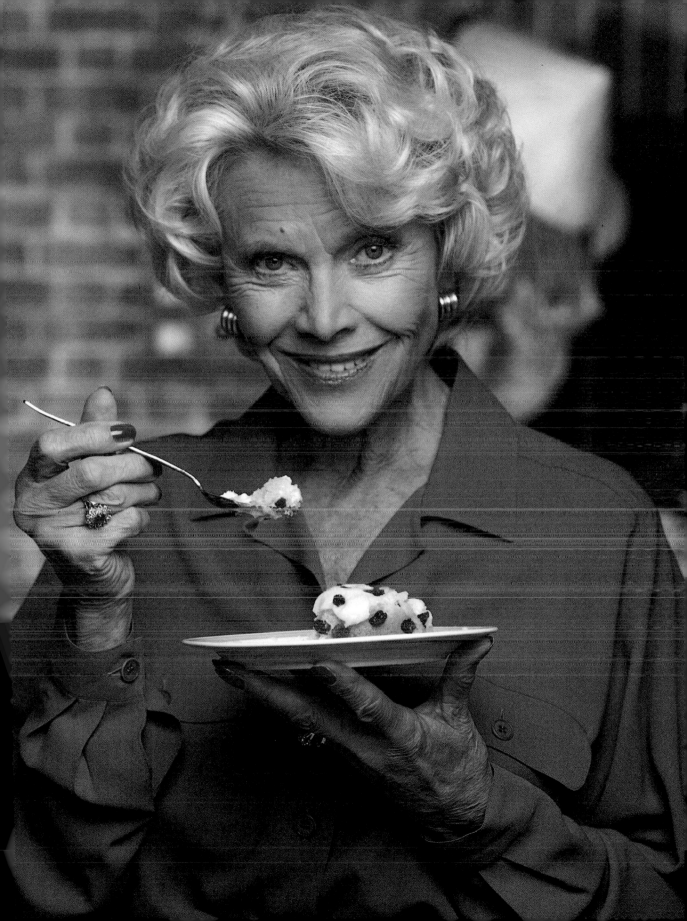

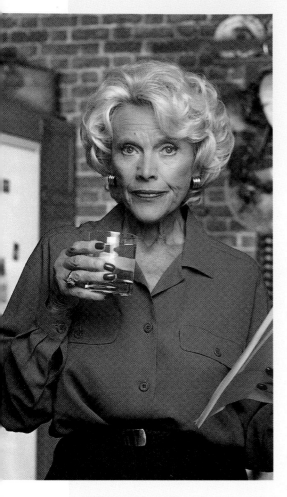

I drink plenty of water
every day and definitely
feel better for it.

be the best of whatever is in season at the time.
- *I adore fresh peas, broccoli and baby cauliflowers, although I'm not too keen on aubergine or cabbage. I think cabbage suffers an image problem with me because my mother overcooked it so often when we were children. We never had vegetables like broccoli or courgette when we were young so they are quite safe.*
- *On the rare occasions when I have a dinner party (and I never invite more than six people) I have a couple of tried and tested recipes which I've mastered and can rely on to turn out perfectly every time. I may not actually enjoy being in the kitchen but when I do cook I am something of a 'Little Miss Perfectionist' so I always want everything to be just right, for the food and the plates to be hot and for all the dishes to be ready at the same time.*
- *As you've heard I've got a grand passion for desserts, so whether I'm entertaining at home or eating out at a restaurant, I'm afraid that a small portion of treacle tart or lemon torte will invariably pass my lips.*

SEVEN DAY HEALTHY EATING PLAN

If you really want to get yourself into shape, the best way to start off is by following a healthy eating plan like the one given here. According to Dr Frank Ryan, an adviser to the Nutrition Institute, if you are planning to go on any sort of balanced diet, you should ensure that you consume around 1,500 calories a day. This will guarantee that you get enough food for energy but will enable you to lose weight too as long as you are taking regular exercise. Make a shopping list of all the things you'll need for the week ahead and don't stray from it. Use our daily suggestions as a guideline for future healthy eating.

Eat the following every day:
- *Unlimited steamed vegetables*
- *Three pieces of fresh fruit*
- *1 diet yoghurt or fromage frais*
- *25g (1oz/1tbsp) low fat spread*
- *420ml ($^3/_4$pt/1$^3/_4$ cups) pint semi-skimmed milk*
- *Tea and coffee with sweetener and milk from the allowance can be taken throughout the day*
- *Low-calorie drinks can be taken freely (although my own preference is for water).*

DAY ONE

BREAKFAST: Bowl of muesli with milk from the daily
   allowance. Glass of orange juice.

LUNCH: One slice of ham in a sandwich made with two small
   slices of brown bread. Piece of fruit from allowance.

DINNER: Mackerel Portuguese (serves 4).

Method:

Split and bone the mackerel. Place them in an ovenproof dish,
season with salt and pepper and squeeze a little lemon juice over
them. Bake for 20–25 minutes in a moderate oven. Meanwhile,
shred the red pepper and chop the onion. Fry both gently in the
olive oil. Add the crushed garlic, paprika and chopped tomatoes
and stir.

   Simmer slowly for about 10 minutes until the mixture is soft,
spoon over the fish and serve with a huge portion of vegetables
from your daily allowance and a baked potato with any left-over
spread.

   Follow with a portion of fresh fruit from allowance.

Ingredients:

4 mackerel

salt and pepper

lemon juice

red pepper

$^1/_2$ onion

1 tbsp olive oil

1 clove garlic, crushed

1 tsp paprika

175g (6oz/$^3/_4$ cup) chopped tomatoes

DAY TWO

BREAKFAST: Boiled egg with 2 slices of toast and 2 teaspoons
   of marmalade. Cup of tea.

LUNCH: Wholemeal bap filled with slice of turkey, mixed salad
   and two sliced medium-sized tomatoes. Yoghurt from
   allowance.

DINNER: Spicy Chicken (serves 4).

Method

Mix the olive oil with the clear honey, curry powder, mustard
and salt and pepper. Pour the sauce over chicken drumsticks and
place in a moderate oven for an hour, turning once. Serve with
boiled rice. (Make it brown rice if possible.) Follow with fruit
from allowance.

Ingredients

2 tbsp good olive oil

100g (4oz/$^1/_2$ cup) clear honey

1 tsp curry powder

4 tbsp ($^1/_4$ cup) German mustard
   (or wholegrain)

salt and pepper

12 skinned chicken drumsticks

DAY THREE

BREAKFAST: Serving of All Bran. One slice of toast and a cup
   of tea.

LUNCH: Baked potato with small tin of baked beans (reduced

sugar and salt) and crunchy salad. Yogurt from allowance.
DINNER: Cod Provençale (serves 4).

Ingredients:

4 cod steaks, approximately
      100g (4oz) each
lemon juice
salt and pepper
1 tbsp olive oil
1 green (bell) pepper, chopped
      and deseeded
1 onion, chopped
3 sticks celery, chopped
175g (6oz/^{3}/$_{4}$ cup) chopped tomatoes
1 clove garlic, crushed
pinch of fresh oregano, chopped
175g (6oz/1^{1}/$_{2}$ cup) sliced
      mushrooms

Method

Wash and dry the cod steaks, place in a shallow ovenproof dish and sprinkle with lemon juice and pepper.

Heat the olive oil in a frying pan and lightly fry the green (bell) pepper, onion and celery. Stir in the chopped tomatoes, the garlic, and a pinch of salt and oregano.

Bring to the boil and simmer for 10 minutes.

Add the sliced mushrooms and simmer for a further 5 minutes. Pour the vegetables over the fish, cover with foil and cook in a preheated oven at 180°C (350°F/Gas Mark 4) for 30–40 minutes. Serve with extra vegetables, a large baked potato and a glass of dry wine. Finish with fresh fruit from allowance.

DAY FOUR

BREAKFAST: Two Weetabix with milk from allowance. Glass
    of fresh orange juice.
LUNCH: Big bowl of fresh vegetable soup, two slices of toast
    and yoghurt from allowance.
DINNER: Salmon Salsa (serves 4).

Ingredients

1 red onion
1 green chilli
1 red chilli
2 tsp good olive oil
splash of balsamic vinegar
4 pieces of (boneless) salmon fillet
      (approximately 100g/4oz
      each)
4 sprigs of fresh dill

Method

Make a salsa by finely chopping the red onion, green chilli and red chilli. (Make absolutely sure you remove all the seeds from the chillies as these are very hot.) Add the olive oil and a splash of balsamic vinegar. Allow to stand for 30 minutes.

Microwave the salmon fillets and garnish them with sprigs of dill and the salsa sauce. Serve with vegetables from allowance and a large portion of pasta, something like fusilli is perfect.

DAY FIVE

BREAKFAST: One toasted wholemeal muffin, tea and yoghurt
    from allowance.
LUNCH: Mix 75g (3oz/^{1}/$_{2}$ cup) of tuna in brine (drained) with
    4 walnut halves, chopped, and black pepper. Shred some

lettuce and cucumber and pile the tuna mix on top. Serve with two rice cakes.

DINNER: Chinese Chicken (serves 4).

Method

Heat the sunflower oil in a heavy based wok or frying pan and gently stir fry the sliced chicken breasts. Add the sliced onions, sliced mushrooms, sliced celery, bamboo shoots and garlic. Mix together the tomato purée (paste), sherry and soya sauce and add to the pan (add a little extra water if necessary). Heat through and serve with 175g (6oz/1 cup) of wild rice. One glass of wine. Follow with fruit from allowance.

Ingredients

4 tbsp (¼ cup) sunflower oil

4 chicken breasts, sliced

2 onions, sliced

175g (6oz/1½ cups) sliced mushrooms

2 celery sticks, sliced

175g (6oz/¾ cup) bamboo shoots

1 clove garlic, crushed

2 tbsp each of tomato purée (paste), sherry and soya sauce

DAY SIX

BREAKFAST: Two Shredded Wheat with milk from allowance. Glass of juice and cup of tea.

LUNCH: Piece of cold, grilled (broiled) chicken with skin removed, large salad (some supermarkets now sell fat free dressings) and wholemeal bap.

DINNER: Saffron Risotto (serves 4).

Method

Heat 2 tablespoons of vegetable oil in a heavy-based pan and add the arborio (risotto) rice, well-washed, stirring in gradually. Add the cardamom seeds and cashew nuts before pouring in the water. Add the peas and salt to taste. Mix the ingredients together and then cover. Cook slowly for 20 minutes. In a separate pan, gently stir-fry the onion, red (bell) pepper and mushrooms in the remaining oil until soft. Add the saffron milk to the rice. Drain the stir-fried vegetables on kitchen paper and add them to the pan also, along with the prawns (shrimp). Stir well and cook briefly until heated through. Follow with fruit from allowance.

Ingredients

4 tbsp (¼ cup) vegetable oil

225g (8oz/1½ cup) arborio (risotto) rice

2 crushed cardamom seeds

1 tbsp cashew nuts

350ml (12 fl oz/1½ cups) water

225g (8oz/1 cup) peas

salt

1 small onion, chopped

1 red (bell) pepper, de-seeded and chopped

a handful of mushrooms, sliced

½ tsp saffron filaments, pre-soaked in 2 tbsp milk from allowance

50g (2oz/⅓ cup) cooked prawns (shrimp)

DAY SEVEN

BREAKFAST: Bowl of All Bran with milk from allowance. Cup of tea. Toasted muffin.

LUNCH: Two slices of wholemeal toast with a 227g (8oz) carton of low-fat cottage cheese, large salad and glass of fruit juice.

DINNER: Easy Casserole (serves 4).

Ingredients

1 tbsp sunflower oil

1lb (450g/2 cups) lean, cubed
　braising steak

1 small onion, chopped

225g (8oz/2 cups) sliced
　mushrooms

100g (4oz/²/₃ cup) chopped
　fennel

1 glass red wine

300ml (¹/₂ pt/1¹/₄ cups)
　vegetable stock

1 bouquet garni

salt and pepper

1 tbsp plain (all-purpose) flour

Method

Heat the sunflower oil in a frying pan and fry the braising steak until brown. Add the chopped onion and sliced mushrooms and cook until lightly browned. Add the chopped fennel, red wine, vegetable stock and bouquet garni, and season with salt and pepper.

Place all of the ingredients in a casserole dish with a tight-fitting lid and cook in a moderate oven for 2 hours. Blend the flour with a little water, add to the casserole and return to the oven for a further 15–20 minutes. Serve with heaps of fresh vegetables. Finish with fruit.

Crash diet

If you want to lose weight and remain healthy you should consider healthy eating and a sensible diet to be a long-term commitment. Don't ever crash diet. Think positively and don't weigh yourself every day. To see how you are doing it's best to take a weekly overview.

Fat for life

Fat is often treated with contempt by seasoned dieters but it's important to remember that there are both good and bad fats.

'Don't stop eating fat altogether – it's a natural food and you need a certain amount for normal health,' says Dr Frank Ryan. 'What we all need to do is cut down on the number of foods which contain saturated fat such as full cream milk, lard, cheese spreads, fast food, coconut oil and palm oil.'

For my part I always trim the white fat off any red meat and avoid the skin of goose, duck, chicken and turkey. Cutting down on foods which are high in cholesterol is a good idea too and these include liver, eggs, fish roe and kidney.

FAVOURITE FOODS

There are two types of food in my diet which I'm absolutely passionate about: fish and fibre. Fish is one of my favourite foods and I could eat it for every meal. I

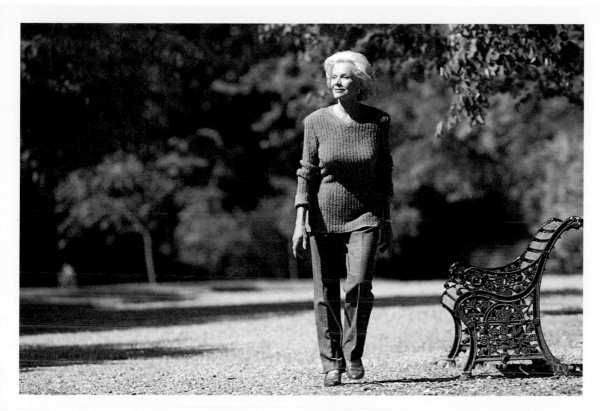

find one of the easiest ways to cook it is in the microwave — from salmon to swordfish it comes out succulent every time. Often, if I get in very late from work I'll simply microwave a piece of fresh fish in minutes and eat it with a hunk of bread. There is truly nothing simpler

Just like fibre, fish is vitally important for women's health. Scientists report that more and more women are now suffering from heart attacks and fish is one of the main foods which helps prevent heart disease. In particular, oily fish like herring and mackerel act by reducing the danger of blood clots in arteries narrowed by cholesterol deposits. Dr Frank Ryan suggests that women should eat oily fish or take two teaspoons of cod liver oil a day. 'Fish oil works by breaking down the levels of saturated fat,' he says. Less oily fish like cod or haddock are also good for us if they are cooked in the right way. Poach, steam, grill (broil), microwave or bake fish. Make fish and chips a very occasional treat and always cook with oils that are high in polyunsaturates — such as corn, soya and sunflower oil. Try virgin olive oil or walnut oils on salads.

Getting fit for life means balancing what we eat with the amount of exercise we take.

Fibre providers

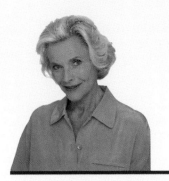

I've been an advocate of more fibre in the diet for many years and have worked alongside Kelloggs in their ongoing campaign to get us all to eat more. It was seeing a close relative suffer from stomach cancer which got me involved with the Colon Cancer Campaign charity and I now do what I can to help them. Fibre has been described as nature's very own vacuum cleaner. It's recommended that we should all eat 18 grams a day and by eating a high-fibre breakfast, for example, you'll keep your weight down, keep hunger at bay and help to clear your system out.

'Eating fibre doesn't have to be boring; it's present in rice, bran, baked beans, fruit and vegetables.'

Fibre is found in a whole host of foods from breakfast cereals and vegetables to fruits and pulses. I'm not the kind of person who will remember to soak beans overnight or prepare a slow-cooked bean casserole but I love lentil soup, broad beans and baked beans and there's plenty of fibre in all of them.

Taken as wheatbran, for example, fibre helps to protect us from bowel disorders including irritable bowel syndrome, piles (haemorrhoids), hernias and constipation by quickening the elimination of waste from the body. There has also been a suggestion, resulting from new research, that a diet rich in wheatbran may also reduce the risk of breast cancer.

I find that if I eat a balanced diet which contains the required 18 grams of fibre a day I rarely get hungry in between meals because the fibre fills me up.

How to include more fibre

- *Don't skip on breakfast. If you don't eat something healthy first thing you will miss out on essential nutrients and these are not made up during the day.*
- *Increase your intake of all kinds of vegetables, especially pulses such as beans and lentils.*
- *Eat more fruit, as snacks or dessert.*
- *Eat more baked beans — they contain 5 grams of fibre per serving compared to 2.6 grams for two slices of brown bread or 1.4 grams for a portion of brown rice.*
- *When out shopping, look for high-fibre versions of your usual foods.*

> *Opt for brown rice, wholewheat pasta and wholemeal bread.*
> • *Drink lots of water (doctors recommend at least 1.2 litres (2pt/5 cups) a day). This will help the fibre to bulk and do its work.*

Organic

There are now some excellent shops selling organic produce all around the country. Two near me, Planet Organic and Wild Oats, specialize in the freshest organic food available which has all been produced without the aid of artificial fertilizers and growth hormones.

From meat and fish to fruits and grains it's now possible to buy almost everything from organic stores, including baby foods. Who knows what the longterm effects of the hormones and antibiotics now being pumped into everything from chicken to pork will have on our health and upon the health of our children? The shiny apples that you see in most shops aren't that way naturally – most have been sprayed with wax.

Although organic food does tend to be a little bit more expensive than mass produced varieties and individual pieces of fruit may not look as perfect as those uniform apples and oranges we see in the high street, I do always try to buy organic food whenever I can.

Not only is the taste better but I like to think that I'm not polluting my body with unnecessary additives. Most supermarkets now have an organic counter within their fruit and vegetable departments and I think the produce is certainly worth trying.

'People get so used to eating the tasteless, mass-produced rubbish that many supermarkets display that when they try organic produce they

Get real: organic foods taste as they should because they are not 'assisted' by anything chemical.

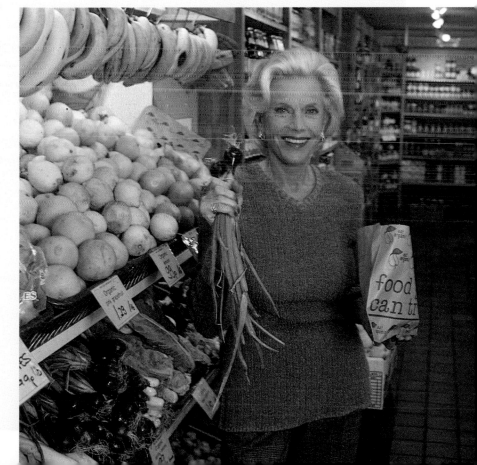

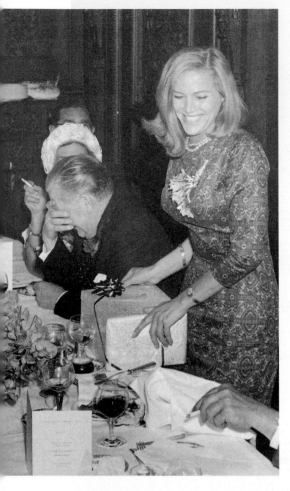

Lunch was lovely and who minds a present with pudding? The gift was a silver fruit dish, by the way!

can't believe the difference in taste,' says Jonathan Dwek of Planet Organic.

Organic produce lost its brown rice and sandals image long ago. Today customers interested in organic goods are of all ages and from all walks of life. As food scares continue and people become more environmentally aware, organic food is the food that consumers are naturally turning to because they trust it.

It's a belief that's certainly endorsed by Stephen Mosbacher of Wild Oats. 'Organic food does tend to be a little more expensive because it's so labour intensive,' says Stephen, 'but it's all a case of supply and demand. As more and more consumers realize that organic food is healthier, so we'll be able to produce more and make it more widely available.'

Eating out

When visiting a restaurant I tend to eat the same sorts of things – fish, pasta, chicken or casseroles – only cooked in ways I could never hope to achieve in my own kitchen. I love starters and I love desserts almost more than I enjoy the main course. I sometimes wish I could have two starters and two puddings.

Occasionally I'll go with a friend to a restaurant and we'll have Chinese or Indian food. I adore Indian food as rice is a particular favourite of mine – it's full of fibre, which is a plus.

Indian food does tend to be fairly calorie-laden but I find that by sticking to dishes that aren't floating in heavy sauces or choosing rice and vegetables that haven't been cooked in ghee it is possible to enjoy the spicy taste without damaging the waistline too much.

I'm not actually capable of eating a great quantity of food – I think it's because I grew up during the war. I have a very healthy appetite but it does alarm me when I see the mountains of food that some people can get through in one sitting.

I've found that the best trick is to eat slowly and savour each mouthful. It takes a little while for the brain to register that the stomach is full, so it is wise to wait at least 20 minutes after eating your main course before considering a pudding. Who knows, you may not feel like it after the wait.

Fast food

One of my rare but loveliest indulgences is fish and chips. I adore them, and they always taste so much better smothered with salt and vinegar straight out of the paper. I know that the batter isn't terribly healthy but sometimes I have the excuse of not being able to eat anything else. For example, the best and almost the only time for indulging in this treat is when I've just come off stage from performing my one-woman show. When I'm appearing in the theatre it's impossible for me to eat before going on stage – my nervous tummy simply won't allow it. Therefore, when the show is over I am absolutely ravenous. Since there are no restaurants open wonderful William Blezard my accompanist, Tano my manager and I sit in the car and steam up the windows as we consume our fish and chips. The car smells for the next week – what glamour!

Apart from fish and chips I'm proud to say that I've never eaten a take-away meal in my life. I've successfully resisted the temptation to try soggy burgers and home-delivered pizzas and can't say I've missed them in the slightest. What could be faster than plunging fresh pasta in boiling water and serving it tossed in extra virgin olive oil with some Parmesan cheese grated on top? Or stir-frying a selection of chopped vegetables and adding some rice noodles?

Those are much healthier, cheaper and quicker options than waiting for a pizza-delivery man to turn up. Try grilling strips of seasoned chicken and serving them on top of a dish of lightly dressed rocket and lettuce leaves tossed with a handful of pine nuts for a delicious warm salad. Or, buying a pack of fresh gnocchi (potato dumplings) from the supermarket and serving it with sweet tomatoes, roughly chopped and heated through in a saucepan with fresh basil leaves. It beats a soggy take-away pizza with a riot of toppings any day. I have nothing against restaurant pizzas, but fast food is not for me.

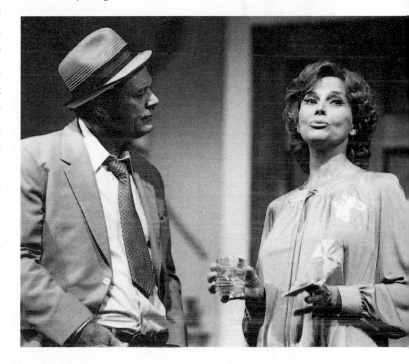

Here I am on stage in Perth. The 'whisky' in my hand is actually cold tea and quite foul.

TEN ESSENTIAL MOOD FOODS

Certain foods have a particularly beneficial effect on our health. How many times have you eaten a fat- and calorie-laden cream tea or Christmas dinner only to feel like death all afternoon and other times felt that you could run a marathon after consuming a crunchy salad and dish of fresh fruit? I know that I feel alive and somehow cleaner when I've eaten particular foods. So it seems logical to me that if something feels like it's doing me good, it probably is. Here's how I eat myself to health:

- *GARLIC: This pungent vegetable is an essential part of my diet. It is thought to combat yeasts in the gut and may limit the rise in cholesterol after a heavy meal. Therefore, it may prevent heart attacks.*

- *LEAFY VEGETABLES: Greens and spinach are rich in folic acid, potassium and iron and may help fight against birth defects and heart disease.*

- *OILY FISH: Eaten twice a week, oily fish like mackerel and herring will help reduce the level of saturated fat.*

- *CARROTS: Along with CANTALOUPE MELON and SWEET POTATOES, carrots are thought to help protect against cancer of the breast, stomach and lungs.*

- *BANANAS: As well as being an instant energy booster, bananas contain potassium, which is thought to lower blood pressure.*

- *ONION: Eaten raw, onion is said to help the levels of 'good' cholesterol (HDL) to keep the arteries clear. OLIVE OIL is another food which actively boosts 'good' cholesterol.*

- *OATBRAN: A tablespoon of oatbran a day helps lower the levels of 'bad' cholesterol (LDL). The peptin contained in APPLES will also do something similar.*

- *BRUSSELS SPROUTS: Along with broccoli, this vegetable is thought to be capable of preventing the growth of tumours.*

- *YOGHURT: Live yogurt is excellent for replacing 'good' bacteria in the gut as well as helping to treat thrush.*

- *SHELLFISH: Prawns (shrimp), lobster and mussels are all high in zinc. Not only is this supposed to be an aphrodisiac but seafood also provides selenium, low levels of which have been linked to cancer.*

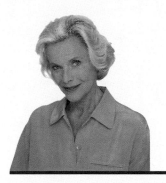

'Who could live without garlic? Certainly not me, and it is also wonderfully beneficial to the health.'

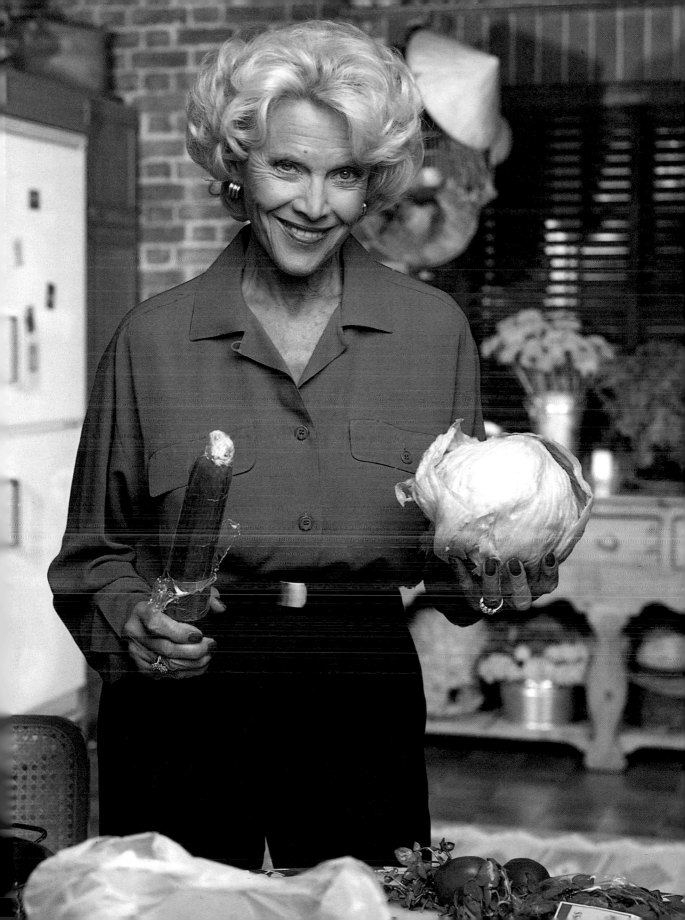

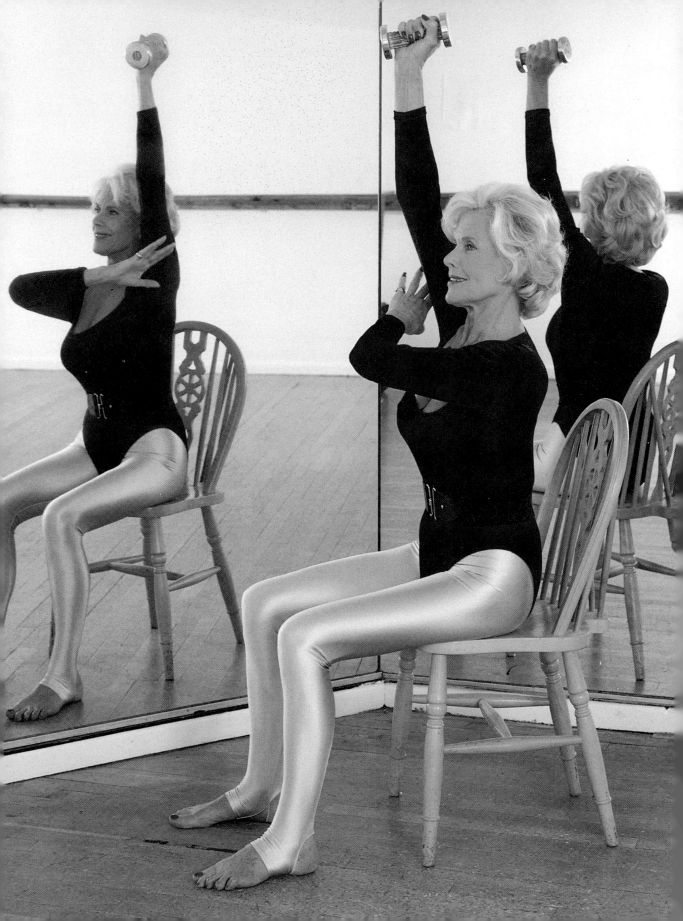

SHAPING UP AND STEPPING OUT

It's over 30 years since I threw and thwacked my way through *The Avengers* but the action image has stuck. My love of exercise and fighting probably comes from my father, who made us walk for miles and taught me how to box at four. It came about when my brother Ken was bullied one time too many and my father decided that he needed to know how to defend himself and whatever Ken did, I did. Father rigged up a pillow as a punch bag and he taught us exactly where to aim on the chin. According to my mother I knocked out two older boys in defending Ken over the years. The thought of my violence obviously shocked me so much that I've blocked it out of my mind, but I do remember knocking out Peter Middleton, a boy at school, when he tried to take my skipping rope.

Winning was always very important to my father. He was not content that I was the games captain at Ealing Secondary School; since I could win the running forwards race I had to win the running backwards race too – quite a feat. My father believed that you had to 'bleed for it'. He always said it was a quotation from Noel Coward, that success was something that required that kind of sacrifice, but it sounds a little too earthy to be Coward for me.

Consequently, when the creators of *The Avengers* suggested I learn judo for the part of Cathy Gale I wasn't in the slightest bit fazed, though, of course, I said I must be taught. I got my first throw in during the third episode and I had had no proper judo training whatsoever. A fellow actor – perversely enough called De'Ath – showed me how to do a very simple throw and the director loved it, although I'm not so sure the actor did. From then on judo fights were included in every episode.

CONTENTS

I fondly imagined that I would be given private judo lessons and was horrified when I went down the basement stairs of a gym run by the Robinson Brothers to find a dozen male bodies sweating on the mats. Because I was going where no woman had gone before I was shoved behind a curtain to change and found myself at eye level with a line of grotty jockstraps. It was full of charm.

I actually took to judo very well and became quite good at it, getting to brown belt level, but the action on screen wasn't without its own drama.

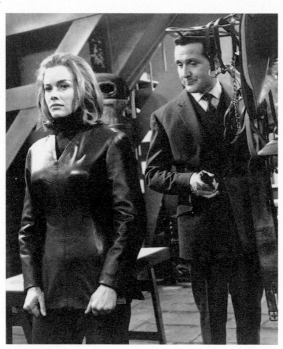

The Avengers. Just look at that hard floor – no wonder my back suffered from all those judo throws.

One time, I was shooting a scene with the wrestler Jackie Pallo. We were fighting next to an open grave and the idea was that I should kick him in the face, grab a spade, he would try to wrest it from me, then I would let go and he would fall into the grave. We had run through this five times for the cameras and were both utterly exhausted when the director called for us to do it again. I was on a hillock and Jackie was on a lower level. I was supposed to put my boot on his face and push. Unfortunately in my haste I grabbed the shovel and, realizing my mistake, turned and kicked Jackie full in the face. Although his eyes completely crossed, he miraculously managed to get up to my level and fight me for the shovel before falling backwards into the grave unconscious. I felt absolutely dreadful and wailed 'I'll never fight again', but he finally came round and of course I did.

Jackie wasn't the only casualty resulting from my judo – I suffered because of it too. Lacking a decent-sized bottom I frequently used to land on the base of my spine, particularly when doing stomach throws, and as the studio's cement floor was covered in neither carpets nor mats, I've suffered from a bad back ever since.

However, it was a chance conversation with a dancer during a production of *The Sound of Music* in which I was starring that led me to Pilates, a form of exercise which has now transformed my life.

Similar in many ways to the Alexander Technique or T'ai Chi, Pilates is a non-aerobic method of exercise that works by lengthening and stretching all the major muscle groups in a balanced way.

Pilates has helped my back enormously and when I've been to a class I feel a foot taller and wonderfully well. Usually it's taught on a one-to-one basis but with the guidance of my teacher, the Pilates expert Alan Herdman, we've devised a way for you to do it at home too.

HOW TO APPROACH EXERCISE

Motivating ourselves to do any form of exercise is inevitably a chore. I can always think of a million and one other things I could or should be doing rather than getting on with the important business of staying in shape.

Whether you're a busy mum or a high-powered executive, there never seems to be a time when you're not committed to something else or totally exhausted from simply getting through the day, does there? But being fit is important. No one expects you to become an Olympic athlete overnight but by taking regular exercise you'll find that you will be much more able to cope with a busy life, have more energy and be generally healthier. Experts advise that we should take moderate exercise five times a week or involve ourselves in an energetic activity three times a week. That can mean anything from walking the dog to spring-cleaning the bedroom.

TOP TIPS

1. Vigorous housework, like cleaning the windows or hoovering, can help you keep fit.

2. Walk or cycle to the shops instead of taking the bus (but get the bus back – no one expects you to stagger home with all the shopping!).

3. If you take the bus or tube to work, then get off one stop earlier. (Put your best shoes in a bag and wear some practical walking shoes to get about in.)

4. Take the dog for a brisk walk.

5. Use the stairs instead of a lift or escalator.

6. Do more in the garden. Gardening is a great form of exercise because it involves lifting and stretching. The latest research from the USA suggests that planting and raking are on a par with brisk walking, while shovelling provides as much of a workout as tennis. Sprucing up your garden also provides a psychological boost, but don't forget to bend your knees and lift properly when you're doing it.

7. Make use of the exercise bikes at your local leisure centre or gym.

If you do enough to get slightly out of breath for 20 minutes, three days a week, you'll really feel the benefits. According to the Department of Health, regular activity keeps you supple and less prone to aches and pains. It improves your circulation – so you are less likely to get heart disease, high blood pressure or diabetes – and helps you to relax. And because activity burns off fat and builds muscle, you'll look better too. Physical fitness is made up of three distinct elements, flexibility, strength and endurance, and developing all three is the key to overall well-being. If you seriously want to get into shape then you have to show some commitment.

- *Check with your doctor first to ensure that you are well enough to start a new physical regime.*
- *Find out about cheap exercise classes or women's swimming sessions at your local leisure centre.*
- *Set yourself realistic targets.*
- *Build up gently, forget about 'going for the burn'. If the exercises hurt then stop.*

As well as taking some form of formal exercise, at a fitness club or gym for example, there are also plenty of ways you can get fit in everyday life too.

AEROBIC EXERCISE

Not to be confused with aerobic exercise classes, aerobic exercise includes swimming, fast walking, cycling and skipping. If you perform heartbeat-raising exercise such as this non-stop for at least 12 minutes, it is described as aerobic. The benefit of this is that aerobic exercise is the best type of activity for improving your general level of fitness. It will help your lungs, heart and muscles to perform better.

WOMEN AND EXERCISE

As we get older our bones begin to thin and it's vital for every woman who wants to avoid the ravages of osteoporosis to maintain physical fitness. We actually start losing bone mass at the age of 35, so it's important for women in their thirties, forties and onwards to be active because weight-bearing exercise such as brisk walking, walking up and down stairs and cycling helps to keep our bones strong. Studies show that doing this kind of activity for about half an hour three times a week can keep bones strong and even build them.

According to Diana Moran, TV's former Green Goddess, who wrote a book about beating osteoporosis through diet and exercise, even simple things like hopping on one foot or carrying shopping bags (make sure that the weight is balanced on each side) have bone-boosting effects. One test I would advise for all women approaching 40 is one which checks bone density. I helped to publicize the arrival of one of the first bone density machines at St George's Hospital in Tooting some time ago. Fortunately I was given the all clear but its a good preventative step that all women can take if their local hospital has such equipment.

CYCLING

As well as doing my Pilates exercises I also have an exercise bike in my home. I use it three times a week for 20 minutes and 5 to 12 minutes on other days. Cycling in general is a very good way to get fit because it is a gentle exercise and does not put too much strain on any of the joints. Using an exercise bike is particularly good for me as it means I can exercise in the comfort of my own home at any time, without the worry of pollution or dangerous drivers! Most gyms have them too if you aren't prepared to invest in one yourself.

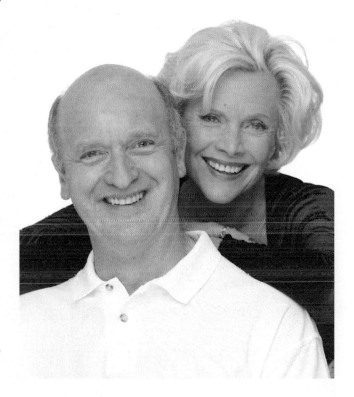

Myself and Alan Herdman, my Pilates instructor.

The bike's control dials also tell me how much effort I am exerting. (Many bikes reveal exactly how many calories one has used up, too.) When you cycle at home, always make sure the room is well ventilated and that your leg is slightly bent when the pedal is furthest away from you.

WALKING

Walking is a great way to get fit too. You can do it anywhere at any time, and it's free. Only this is one area of this book, dear reader, where I suggest you DON'T follow my example.

I had a medical check and although the doctor said I was in very good health he said he thought it might be a good idea if I got some aerobic exercise. I think he was only trying to justify his fee! I said 'If you think I'm going to leap around in an exercise class then forget it', but he said you don't have to jump around, you can just walk very fast as it's the perfect way to get your heartbeat up. Do it for 20 minutes, three times a week.

So, being the obsessive I am, I started walking EVERY day. I have these beautiful gardens opposite my home, but the paths have big impacted stones and as it was autumn and rather slippery I hit a big stone, fell and took almost my entire elbow off. The wound was awful but it didn't stop me walking. Then I went on holiday, came back and a week later did exactly the same thing on the other elbow. At this point my children suggested it might be safer all round if I invested in an exercise bike.

Despite my bad experiences I'm still really hot on walking. Always wear comfortable clothes and trainers, start at a slow pace and gradually build up your speed and distance. You should walk fast enough to become a little breathless and slightly tired but still be able to chat. Hit the ground with your heel first and then roll through the foot to the toe, swinging your arms loosely in rhythm, using opposite arms to legs.

SWIMMING

If you don't like getting hot and sweaty through exercise then swimming is perfect. Start slowly and gradually build up the number of lengths you can do at a time without stopping for a break at each end.

If you aim to swim continuously for 20 minutes then you'll soon begin to feel the effects. As with all exercise, perform it every other day so that your muscles will get a chance to recover in between.

I'm still as fit as I was in *The Avengers*.

STRETCHING

Fitness experts know how important it is to stretch before and after doing any form of exercise. Just as we see Olympic standard athletes stretching their arms and legs before they run or swim, so we should do the same. There's nothing more guaranteed to produce aches and pains than working cold muscles. If you are going for a brisk walk then warm up by marching on the spot for a couple of minutes before you get going. The Pilates exercises which follow are perfect for really elongating and stretching the muscles.

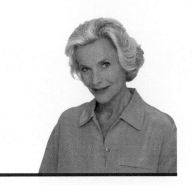

'You'll never find me in an aerobics class. I like controlled exercise – that's why Pilates is good for me.'

FACE EXERCISES

As well as exercising my body I also exercise my face. Someone once showed me a video of face exercises called Facial Workout by Eva Fraser (Virgin) heaven knows if they do any good but as I believe that toning the muscles in the rest of the body is a good idea it must, I feel, follow that it helps the face too. The idea is that you make a lot of terrible faces in order to strengthen particular muscles.

I once tried to show them to my friend Dora Bryan and we laughed so much that she ended up howling 'It's too late, it's all too late!'

I suppose I've been doing my face exercises for about five years. Sometimes I'm sitting at the traffic lights and realize I haven't done them for about two days and end up frightening all of the people in the other cars because I look so hideous doing them.

WHAT IS PILATES?

Alan Herdman introduced Pilates into this country in 1970. A former primary school teacher turned dancer, Alan trained in New York and learnt about Pilates there. Based on the teachings of Joseph Pilates, the exercises centre on posture correction and balance. I had had a bad experience with weight training at a local club before I discovered Alan and the Pilates technique suits me perfectly as it is non-competitive and non-aggressive.

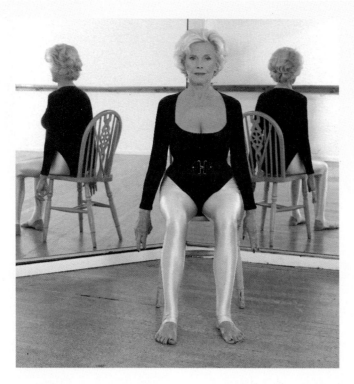

Back to basics: one of the Pilates starting positions. Posture is all, as a straight back brings the body into line.

I hate anything too theatrical and Pilates is unpretentious and nongimmicky, and it works. When I've done a Pilates class I feel I'm walking on air.

In Pilates the emphasis is on posture correction and balance. We do exercises which strengthen the muscle groups and consequently have straighter backs and enjoy a greater feeling of well-being as a result.

The exercises work by strengthening weaker muscles so that the action of each muscle group gradually equalizes. The muscles in the stomach, sides and back are strengthened so that the spine is supported, which, for me, is the most vital part. Unlike aerobics, Pilates does not leave me hot and bothered. Alan believes that 'going for the burn' is one of the worst things we can do.

'The muscles start burning when they're being over-used,' he maintains. 'I want a feeling of wellbeing to be the most important thing. When someone does Pilates properly, their muscles are worked deeply and carefully without exhaustion.'

Pilates is perfect for anyone no matter what their age or their physical condition. Dancers and actors are great devotees of it while many doctors and physiotherapists recommend that stroke victims try it too.

'I've currently got a student who is over 90,' says Alan, 'while many other clients come with their nurses or carers. We've had some great success in helping people back to mobility.' For anyone who suffers from the universal backache, Alan offers hope too. 'In most cases there is nothing wrong with your physique,' he says. 'It's just the way you sit, stand and move that causes the tension to go right down into the lower back. Most people slouch instead of standing tall. The stomach muscles have slackened so that the lower back is much more curved than it should be. That means that the upper torso is also curved and a lot of tension builds up in the shoulders and neck. Simply by strengthening the abdominal area, the tummy, we can support the lower back which helps us to stand up straight.' And when I'm standing straight my body functions correctly and I feel more alert and bright.

Correct breathing is important, too. In Pilates we take a deep breath before each exercise and breathe out on the effort as we are doing the exercise as this helps the muscles to relax.

JOSEPH PILATES

Pilates was devised by a German, Joseph Pilates, over 60 years ago. As a child he suffered from poor health, so in adulthood he was determined to be as strong and fit as possible. He came to Britain just before the First World War and was interned on the Isle of Man, where he developed his fitness plan. There is a story that he also taught his techniques to the other prisoners in his block and that as a result they were strong enough to withstand a bout of flu which wiped out many other men in the camp.

After the war Pilates moved to America and set up a studio in New York. The exercises became popular among dancers and actors and were introduced to Britain when Alan Herdman returned from a trip there in 1970.

What it will do

The wonderful thing about Pilates is that it will actually alter the shape of your body. You won't necessarily lose weight and in some cases you may actually put it on because you will increase the amount of muscle on your body and muscles weigh more than fat. But that's not something to worry about.

Because the muscles are being tightened and firmed your body will become fitter-looking and more shapely. 'I always advise my clients to look at themselves in the mirror rather than agonize on the weighing scales,' says Alan Herdman. 'If you like what you see in the mirror and can get all of your favourite clothes on comfortably, then you're getting there.'

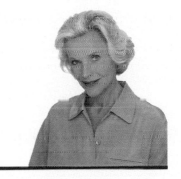

'After a Pilates class I feel wonderfully supple and alert. I walk into the street feeling a foot taller.'

However, just like anything else that's worth having, getting fit through Pilates is hard work. Concentration is all and each exercise has to be worked through 5–10 times. The work is physically tough but the results are sensational.

In a Pilates studio there are no classes where everybody leaps around together in a sweaty mass; each individual has a personl programme and the exercises are done with only quiet classical music playing in the background. Alan believes that one of the major problems with exercise in general is that it's not graded enough. 'Too many people try to do too much, too soon. They join a gym and then get a guilt trip when it doesn't work out. They over-exert themselves or pull a muscle and immediately think that exercise is not for them and never try to get fit again. With Pilates there is no hiding at the back, the exercises are done with thought and control in a quiet and dignified way. We encourage you to feel at peace with yourself and feel good about your body.'

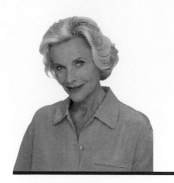

'It's vital to find the time for exercise, however busy you are. Putting it off is all too easy – but coping with a sagging body is not.'

How Pilates fits into my life

At the moment there are not very many Pilates studios around the country although more and more gyms and health clubs are introducing Pilates-based classes. Therefore, what we've done in this chapter is to devise a series of exercises to help you correct posture and balance using Pilates techniques. The aim is to get the muscle groups working as they should and for you to feel as good as I do.

I find it's best to do the exercises every other day on a carpet or rug in my bedroom just before I have my morning shower. It's a time when I'm unhassled and I can just dedicate 10–15 minutes to myself without any outside interruptions. It's not necessary to dress up in a leotard and tights to do them and I often do the buttock squeezes, pulling in the stomach muscles, while I'm standing at the kitchen sink.

With all of the exercises start with 5 and build up to 10 repetitions. Don't be tempted to strain the body and don't forget about the breathing. Remember, in Pilates we breathe out on the effort, which means we breathe out as we actually do the exercise. Given the choice most of us would hold our breath during exercise but correct breathing is essential as it helps you and your muscles to relax.

As with any form of exercise, the exercises won't work to get you fit and slim if you are over-indulging in between. Aim to eat a sensible diet (see Chapter 1) and embrace the concept of a wholly healthy body, inside and out.

MUSCLE NAMES

When you read about any forms of exercises, instructions given will often refer to particular muscles. Here's what they are in simple terms:

- *Hamstrings: muscles from the knee up to the behind*
- *Gluteals: the buttock muscles (in other words the bum)*
- *The abdominals: the tummy*
- *The obliques: part of the tummy muscles*
- *The Latissimus dorsi (or lats): the muscles from the shoulders down towards the pelvis which stabilize the shoulder blades*
- *Biceps: muscles on the front of the upper arms*
- *Triceps: muscles at the back of the upper arms.*

What you'll need

In order to try the exercises at home you'll need a few simple accessories.

1. *A kitchen chair*
2. *A pillow or cushion (for placing between the knees to stop the legs shaking and to place under the tummy to support the lower back)*
3. *A book (to support the back of the head)*
4. *A couple of small fitness weights or cans of soup.*
5. *A small towel (to place under the knees during certain floor exercises).*

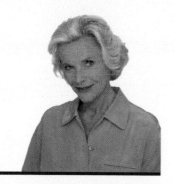

'There's no excuse not to try Pilates. You simply need a few household items and a little determination.'

THE EXERCISES

The exercises in Pilates don't have flashy, gimmicky names. So we've simply numbered them from 1 to 10 and given a short explanation of what the exercise will do for each part of the body.

1. FLOOR EXERCISES

How to start

For the basic starting position for each of the following exercises lie on your back, on the floor. Feet should be flat on the floor with knees parallel and raised to the ceiling about 7.5–10cm (3–4 inches) apart.

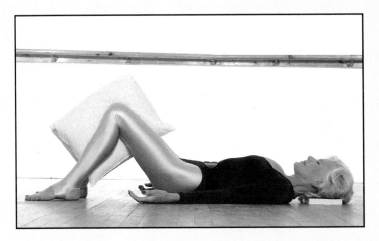

Place a pillow between the knees (to help stabilize the hips and work the inner thighs) and hold it firmly there. Your head should be supported on a paperback book while your arms are by your sides with elbows relaxed and palms facing upwards or downwards, whichever is more comfortable.

How to do it

Get into the mood for exercising by relaxing the body, which should feel heavy on the floor. Feel the length of your spine on the floor too. Neck and shoulders should be relaxed. Breathe in through the nose and as you breathe out through the mouth gently pull the navel down to the spine.

Repeat this 5 times, working up to 10 eventually.

Benefits

This will help you to practise breathing and to find the centre of your torso. You'll feel where your tummy is and gently stretch out the lower back in a passive way.

2. PELVIC TILTS

How to start

Lie on the floor in the same starting position as in exercise one

How to do it

Breathe in and as you breathe out tighten the lower buttock muscles.
Pull in the stomach muscles and slowly curl the lower back off the
floor

Hold the lift to breathe in and as you breathe out slowly take the
spine back down to the starting position.

Benefits

This exercise is to strengthen the pelvic floor muscles and
the lower tummy and tighten the lower buttock muscles.
Basically it will stop your bottom from dropping to
your knees!
Remember, don't think of the back doing the work —
the stomach muscles and lower buttock muscles should
be working here.

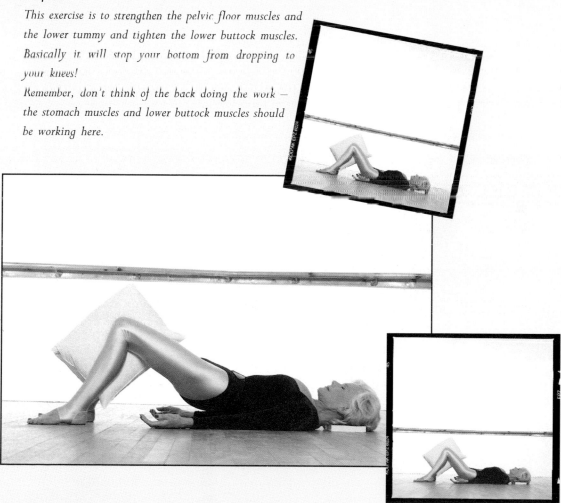

PELVIC TILTS WITH ARMS

How to start

Start in the same starting position on the floor.

How to do it

Next lift the buttocks off the floor as in the previous exercise. From the lift position, as you breathe in, stretch your arms behind your head with the pelvis lifted.

Then, as you breathe out, lower the pelvis to the floor in exactly the same way as in the last exercise, remembering to use the stomach and lower back muscles as you roll down. Slowly stretch your arms along the floor as you are lowering down to elongate the body.

As you breathe in bring your arms back to your sides, returning to the resting position.

Benefits

This will gently stretch and elongate the upper body. Remember, do not lift the pelvis too high and don't arch the back on the way down.

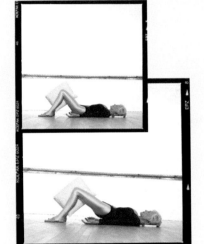

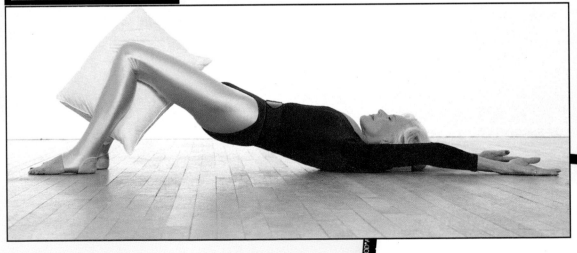

3. BUTTOCKS AND BACKS OF THIGHS

How to start

Lie on the floor, face downwards, with a pillow under your tummy, supporting your back. Fold your arms and rest your forehead on your hands. Keep the legs parallel and straight.

How to do it

Take a breath in and as you breathe out squeeze the buttock muscles together without moving the legs (feel as though you are squeezing a small cushion between your upper thighs).

Hold for about 4 seconds. Relax and breathe in.

This one can be practised standing at the sink or at the bus stop, though upright of course, or people will think you are a little odd. Alternatively, to work the back of the legs, squeeze the buttocks in exactly the same way but as you breathe out slowly bend one knee so that the heel comes up towards the middle of the buttocks

Do this 10 times on one leg and 10 times on the other.

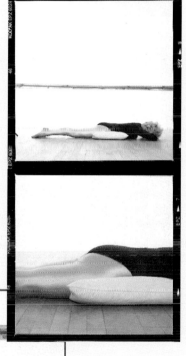

Benefits

These exercises will firm the buttocks and work the back of the thighs and lower tummy muscles to help stabilize the pelvis or hips. Remember, if the bended knee feels uncomfortable put a small pad (a folded towel) between your knee and the floor.

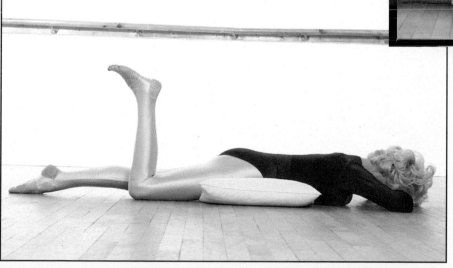

4. INNER THIGHS

How to start

Lie in a straight line on your side, stretch your arm out and rest your head upon it. Bend your top leg onto a cushion in front of you (see the accompanying picture) and put your top hand on your hip (to keep the waistline long). This can be done alongside a wall or a piece of furniture to keep you straight. The bottom leg is parallel and the knee is slightly relaxed.

How to do it

Take a breath in and as you breathe out lift the bottom leg off the floor and hold for 4 counts. Breathe in and lower down.
Return to your original starting position.

Benefits

This exercise will work the wobbly bits on the inner thighs. Remember to pull the tummy in to support the back and keep it in a straight line. Lift the leg up only as high as the hips will allow — if your hips move when you lift your leg you are going too high.

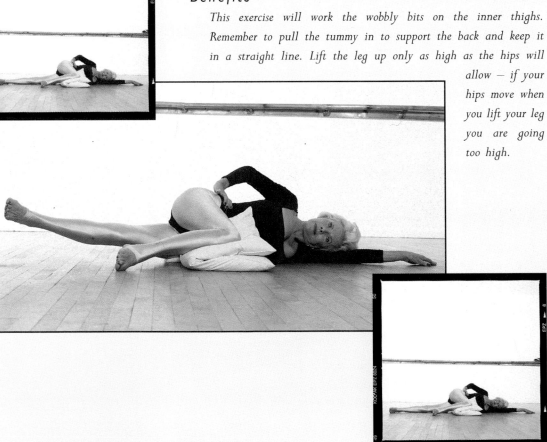

5. TUMMY MUSCLES

How to start

There are two ways to do this exercise and the first gives extra support to the head. Lie on the floor with your feet apart, knees raised to the ceiling and arms behind your head.

How to do it

Breathe in, and as you breathe out lift the upper back and head forward and gently curl your body towards your knees. Repeat 5 times, building to 10.

Relax back to the resting position.

Benefits

These exercises will strengthen tummy muscles which are very important for supporting the lower back. They'll also help flatten the tummy. Remember, as you bring the head forward breathing in, try not to tense the neck. As you reach forward breathing out, soften the rib cage by drawing in the stomach muscles and don't let the hips move. Prevent the tummy muscles from bulging forward by not coming up too far each time and don't be too enthusiastic. Start small and gradually enlarge the movement.

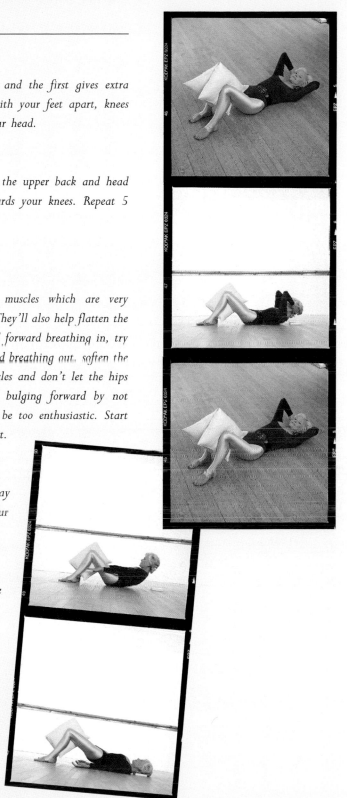

An alternative

Once you've mastered the exercise this way you could also try it with your arms by your side.

How to start

Start in the same position as in the previous exercise (see above).

How to do it

Breathe in and as you breathe out lift the upper back and head forward and gently curl the body and stretch your fingers up towards your knees, reaching forward. Return to our original starting position.

6. SIDE MUSCLES

How to start

Lie on your back with a pillow between your knees.
Put your right hand behind your head (with your elbow about 5cm/2 inches off the floor) and your left hand by your side with the palm facing down.

How to do it

Breathe in and as you breathe out turn towards your left knee, stretch the left hand away and reach your right elbow and shoulder towards your left knee.

An alternative

Put your left hand behind the head, elbow 5cm (2 inches) off the floor. Stretch the right arm across the body diagonally and breathe out as you turn the right hand and shoulder towards the left knee.

Benefits

These exercises work the side muscles which help you move from side to side (the obliques). They will strengthen the muscles around the waist and help trim the waistline. Remember, don't let the knee muscles tighten and if the exercise hurts at all, stop.

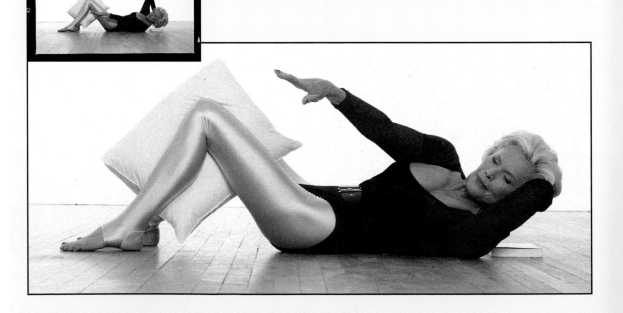

7. THE BACK

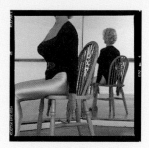

Actors refer to the muscles under the shoulder blades by the curious name of the Colly Curtains because they are reminiscent of the swagged curtains at the London Coliseum. There are three exercises in this sequence.

How to start

Sit on a chair with a straight back. Put both your feet on the floor with the knees at right angles and the tummy pulled in. Your arms should be hanging down by your side with palms facing backwards.

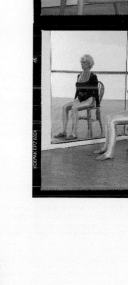

How to do it

Breathe in and as you breathe out, push the palms back behind you. You'll feel the muscles behind the shoulders begin to work. Breathe in and bring the arms back to the starting position

Benefits

These exercises are wonderful for keeping the torso straight, helping to hold the shoulders in place and stopping tension in the neck. Remember, don't let the body sag. Keep the spine upright and pull your navel into the spine. Don't take the arms back too far or the neck will strain.

THE STRESS RELIEVER

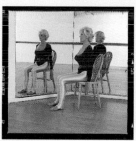

How to start

Sit on your chair in the same starting position but this time tuck your elbows into your rib cage and extend your arms out in front of you with the palms to the ceiling.

How to do it

As you breathe in gently open both arms out to the side. Breathe out and return to the starting position.

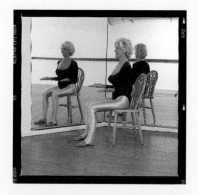

Benefits

This exercise will open out the upper chest, help correct a rounded back and work the muscles around the shoulder blades. Remember to try to keep the elbows tucked into the ribs all the time with arms parallel to the floor. Keep the back straight and you'll find this is a very good stress reliever.

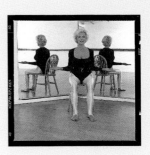

THE COSSACK

How to start

Still sitting on the chair in the same position, fold your arms lightly in front of you. Wrists need to be in line with the breasts.

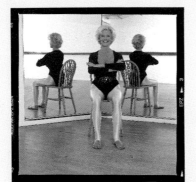

How to do it

Take a breath in and as you breathe out gently turn to the left, taking your left elbow as far round as possible. Breathe in and return to the centre. Breathe out and turn the other way to the right.

Benefits

This exercise will stretch the muscles around the shoulder blades and help to support the neck and the head. Remember, make sure the head and body turn but don't move the pelvis. Keep a straight back and ensure that the elbows lead. Don't let the shoulders lift up, keep them down and don't take them too far round; keep the neck and head comfortable.

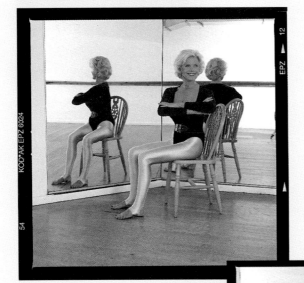

8. ARM EXERCISES WITH WEIGHTS

You'll need your weights or cans of soup for these particular exercises.

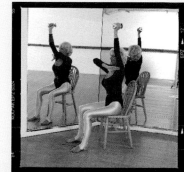

How to start

Sit on the chair again with a straight back. Stretch your left arm straight to the ceiling while holding onto a small weight or can of soup. Take your right arm across the body and support the upper part of the left arm with your right hand. The back of the right hand should be gently pressed against the upper left arm.

How to do it

As you breathe out bend your elbow so that your left hand and weight goes down towards your shoulder.

Breathe in to straighten. Repeat 5 times (building up to 10) and then do the exercise with the other arm.

Return to the starting position

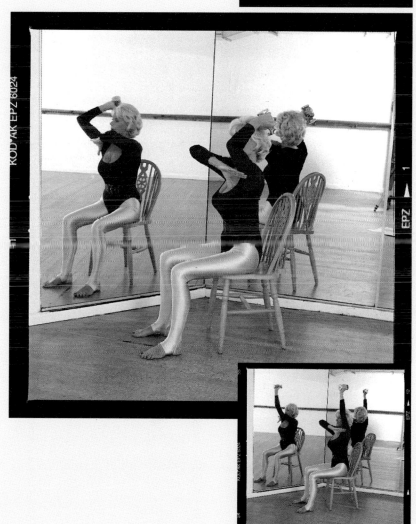

Benefits

This works the unsightly flabby underneath part of your arm. Remember to keep your shoulders as relaxed as possible and keep the sitting posture straight on both sides.

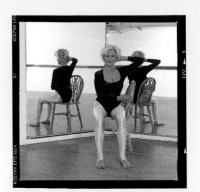

9. SITTING SIDE STRETCHES

How to start

Sit on the side of your chair with your left side against the back of the chair. Place your right hand across the body and gently hold onto the back of the chair, to keep you straight.

How to do it

Place your left hand behind your head, take a breath in and as you breathe out turn your head to the right and gently stretch your left side, elbows first, up to the ceiling and then dip towards the floor so you make a big curve.

Breathe in as you return to the starting position

Do up to 10 on each side.

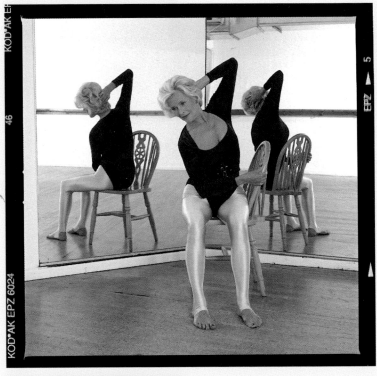

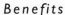

Benefits

This will stretch the waistline right up to the rib cage. Remember to place your hand behind your head so that it is comfortable. Make sure that you are not tense in the neck and don't have your elbow too far back. After each of the exercises on the chair, check that your position is correct, you are not arching your back and your stomach muscles are working.

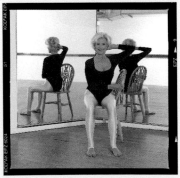

Additional tip

To help to sit up straight put a pillow between the knees and squeeze.

Also, if the chair is not the right height, place something under the feet of the chair so that the position is comfortable.

10. THE BUTTOCKS

How to start

Stand behind the chair, with both feet apart. Hold on to the back of the chair with both hands, standing up very straight.

How to do it

Stretch your left leg out to the side and behind. Place your left hand on your hip to stabilize it. Bend the outstretched leg slightly and lift it off the floor. Hold that position and as you breathe out, lift the bent leg up and down eventually building up to 10 times. Repeat on the other side.

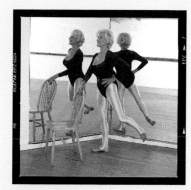

Benefits

This will tone the buttocks. Remember to keep your hips very straight and still and, as with all of these exercises, don't try to do too much too quickly. They may look easy because they don't require an awful lot of physical movement but as with all forms of exercise it's very easy to overdo it.

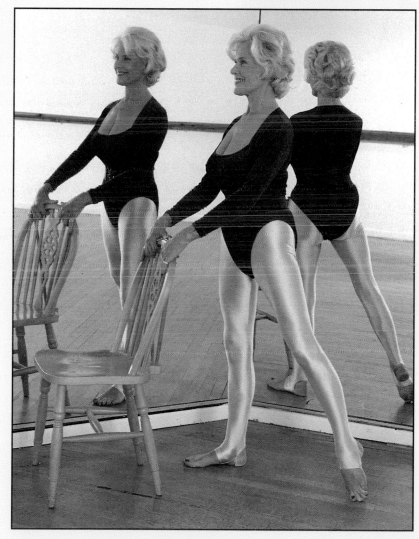

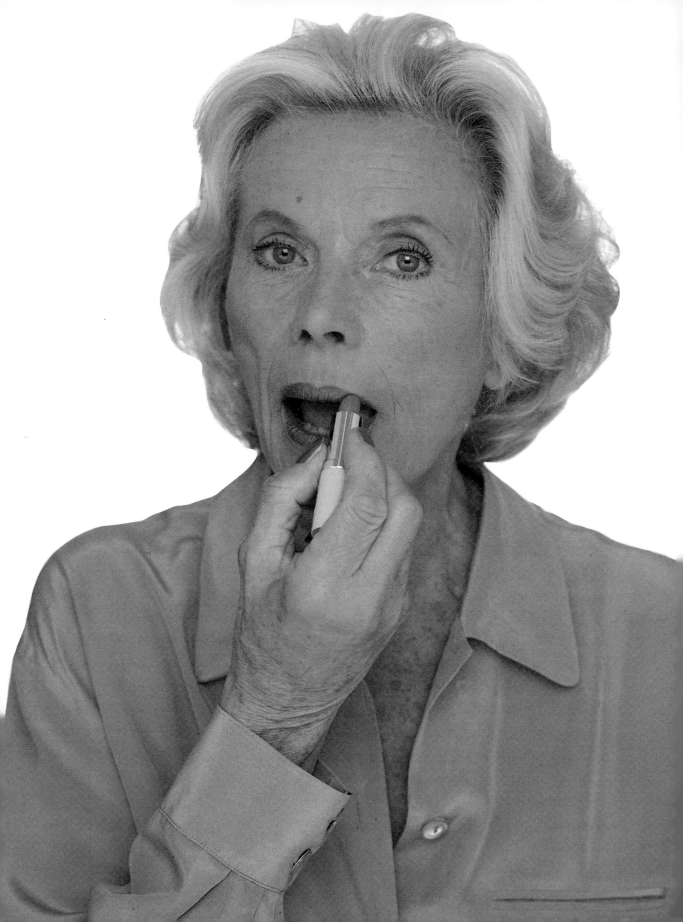

TIPS FROM A TV STAR

There can't be a woman alive who hasn't done something crazy in her life, at least once, in order to make herself more beautiful. I remember reading years ago that dew was good for the skin, so every morning on the way to the studio I'd leap out of the car, scoop up all the dew from the grass and splash it on my face. I doubt if it did any good but it probably made the neighbours smile!

When it comes to beauty my philosophy is simple; I honestly believe that it comes from within. You can slap on all the expensive creams in the world but if you aren't eating a balanced diet and exercizing regularly then you won't get that fresh, healthy glow that to me equates true beauty. I'm lucky in that, like my mother, I have good skin. But everyone has something that's beautiful about them whether it's pretty hair, sexy eyes or a sparkling personality, so it's important to make the most of what you've got and enjoy being yourself. None of us is ever completely happy with the way we look; I've always dreamed of having hair like one of those Pre-Raphaelite beauties but that's never going to happen so there's no point in fretting about it.

The way I look now is, of course, due to basic bone structure plus years of professional advice. I've always thoroughly enjoyed having my face made up by experts on sets from my first film *Fame Is The Spur* through to *The Avengers* and *The Upper Hand*. It's a lovely, indulgent feeling when someone else transforms you.

But like all women I've spent a fortune on products that don't work and on colours that don't suit me and to this day I still can't find the perfect eye liner or maybe I'm just incapable of applying it properly.

CONTENTS

Skin Care • Make-up • Tanning • Nails • Feet • Teeth • Hair • Cosmetic Surgery

One of the most important things I've learnt over the years is the need to treat the skin kindly – it does the skin no good at all to brutalize it. I've spent a career under the glare of hot studio lights and heavy theatrical make-up; I wore glittery cosmetics and false eyelashes in the Sixties and Seventies, but have always been fanatical about cleansing my skin. I've only ever slept in my make-up once and I felt absolutely horrible in the morning. No matter how late I get in or how indulgent I've been I always cleanse, and it's not a chore because it's something I've always done – like cleaning my teeth. If you live in a city, as I do, where pollution is a problem then it's vital to keep the skin scrupulously clean in order for it to breathe and thrive.

What works best for me is not to wash my face at all. In fact, I've not washed my face in 30 years. As my skin tends to be a little dry I prefer to use a creamy cleanser and steer clear of drying soaps.

In the early days of my career in the theatre I used to slap on thick theatrical make-up which came in numbered sticks. The most commonly used ones were five and nine. Nowadays both in TV and in the theatre the actual base is exactly what you would wear in the daytime, although possibly a shade darker in the theatre, so as not to be bleached out by the lights.

Today, modern TV studio lighting and subtle make-up shades mean that my look is far more toned down and natural than when I first started out. I've learned a few tricks along the way – they've worked for me and they may work for you too.

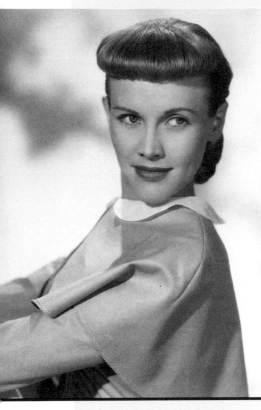

The face of an up and coming actress. 'I looked after my skin meticulously even in the early days.'

SKIN CARE

People constantly ask me how I keep my skin looking so good. Well, the answer is simple – I take care of it. Maintaining my good complexion is essential to me, both privately and professionally. It responds to the care and attention I lavish on it. I believe that moisture is the key to smooth, young-looking skin, but we are what we eat so healthy foods are essential too.

- *Fresh foods provide vital minerals and vitamins.*
- *Whole grains, fruits and vegetables contain the minerals that*

are required for healthy skin.

- *Seeds, nuts, oils like olive oil and green leafy foods provide the fatty acids needed for maintaining supple skin.*

Combining a healthy eating plan with due care and attention is the way to care for the skin.

The top layer of skin which covers our entire bodies is called the epidermis and this is capable of replacing itself if it is damaged or worn away. Skin is our natural barrier against the world but it takes a daily battering. Over 75 per cent of women now claim to have sensitive skin which reacts to factors such as perfume, pollution, sunlight and stress. Dermatologists agree that sunlight is the biggest enemy of the skin and no matter how great you look with a tan (and I know that I feel instantly re-energized when I'm golden brown), remember that skin cancer is on the increase.

Despite the fortunes we spend on expensive cosmetics, I've found that maintaining a daily routine is the best treat I can give my skin.

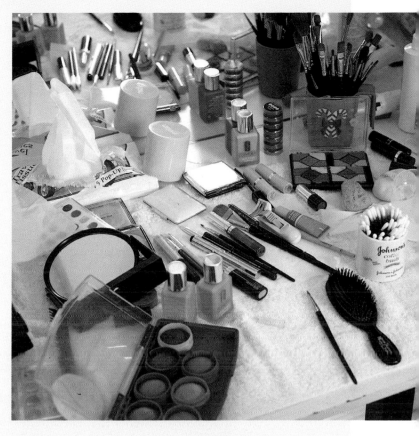

Cleansing

Alll the make-up in the world won't make you look beautiful unless your skin is glowing and for me cleansing is vital. I started work as an actress at 17 and watched people applying my make-up perfectly. But I quickly learnt that being made up at seven in the morning took its toll. In those days, I'd have my hair done, sit under a dryer for an hour and go through the whole day with strong studio lights beating down on me. I jolly well knew that if I didn't clean my face properly at the end of the day the make-up would become embedded.

In this business you come under the scrutiny of people whose job it is to make you look good and they make it very clear if

The Essential Kit:

- Eyelash curler to maximise lashes.
- Eyeshadow brushes — square in shape for control.
- Eye liner brushes — as fine as possible.
- Blusher brush — thick and round to allow blending
- Lipbrush to get into the corners
- Cotton buds for applying, blending or removing.
- Small sponge for applying base.
- Eyelash comb.
- Eyebrow brush.

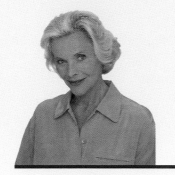

'I prefer the natural colour of my eyes to be the dominating feature, not the eye shadow.'

you are not helping them with the lifestyle you lead. However, I remember one make-up artist at Universal Studios in Hollywood who always managed to convince me that he'd succeeded in making me look more wonderful than the day before by some nuance of make-up and I always left his room feeling fabulously confident. This was a far cry from my mother, who always used to say, 'You'll pass in a crowd.' She was probably determined that I shouldn't become vain.

I've tried all the expensive cleansers on the market and found that one from Boots suits me best. Every night I remove all of my make-up from my face and neck with cream cleanser. I wipe it off at first with tissues and finish off with cotton wool dampened with purified water.

Toner

I don't use a toner or astringent because I find them a little too harsh on my skin. I don't invest in a separate eye make-up remover either because I find a thick, creamy cleanser can take off the lot quite adequately. (Don't ever be tempted to tug at your eyelids when removing shadow and mascara – I know it takes longer to do it gently but you'll be glad you took the time in later life when your skin may not be as elastic as it is now.) This is a routine that suits me and my skin but it obviously won't work for everyone. If your skin is normal to oily then you may prefer to wash it and here one of the many wash-off cleansers available would be ideal. When cleansing any type of skin it's best to work upwards from the neck, taking care not to drag the skin, and keep working the cleanser in until the cotton wool or tissue comes away clean. With a wash-off cleanser you can complete the process by gently dabbing the skin clean with damp cotton wool and splashing with cold water. Even though I don't use toner, many women

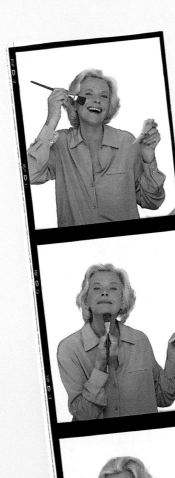

The more natural look is in vogue nowadays; choose your colours carefully to compliment your skin tone.

do find it the perfect way to 'finish off' a cleansing routine by closing the pores and leaving the skin feeling refreshed. Try to find the kindest toner available as I cannot believe that an astringent that stings your skin after use can be good for you. At times when I have found myself without any cleanser I've compromised by using Vaseline or even olive oil, which I've hated – but anything is better than going to sleep still fully made up.

Moisturizer

Moisturizer is vital for women of any age, unless their skin is excessively greasy, and I apply a rich moisturizer night and day.

Applying moisturizer is best done by smoothing it over the skin with your finger tips. Experts say most moisturizers tend to work best if the skin is slightly damp and that includes moisturizing the body and hands too.

Gently avoid the 'T' zone (the area from the forehead down to the nose and chin) if your skin is oily, and blot the skin with a tissue before applying base or powder.

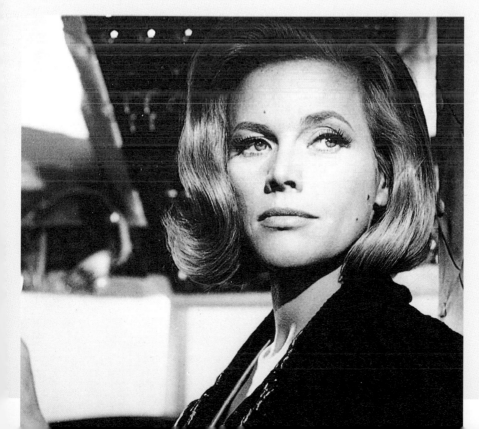

Just look at those false eyelashes . . . the glamour of it all!

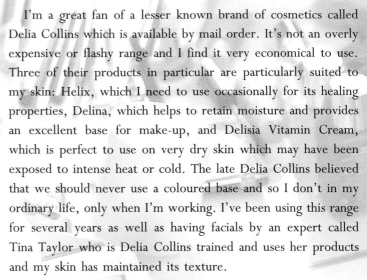

TOP SKIN TIPS

- Don't smoke. Tobacco helps destroy vitamin C which is essential for firm skin.
- Creams containing at least 5 per cent vitamin E may help reduce wrinkles.
- A bad complexion can be made worse by hot weather, excessive alcohol, spicy food and drinks containing caffeine.
- Evening primrose oil capsules, either swallowed or broken and the contents applied to the skin, may help to prevent dry skin.
- Gentle massage can help stimulate sebum production and feed the skin.

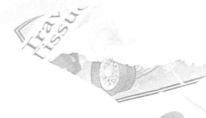

I'm a great fan of a lesser known brand of cosmetics called Delia Collins which is available by mail order. It's not an overly expensive or flashy range and I find it very economical to use. Three of their products in particular are particularly suited to my skin: Helix, which I need to use occasionally for its healing properties, Delina, which helps to retain moisture and provides an excellent base for make-up, and Delisia Vitamin Cream, which is perfect to use on very dry skin which may have been exposed to intense heat or cold. The late Delia Collins believed that we should never use a coloured base and so I don't in my ordinary life, only when I'm working. I've been using this range for several years as well as having facials by an expert called Tina Taylor who is Delia Collins trained and uses her products and my skin has maintained its texture.

Don't forget that many moisturizers now come in tinted varieties so that you don't have to put make-up on top if you don't wish and some also contain an element of sun protection too. Although there is a trend these days to vigorously 'exfoliate' (ie remove any dead skin cells), I try to be as kind to my skin as possible. I avoid harsh scrubs and face masks at all costs and treat the area around my eyes with particular care, never dragging cotton wool or tissues across the skin but instead working from the outside of the eye inwards and always patting the skin dry rather than attacking it with a dry towel.

My essential products

- *Lashings of cream cleanser*
- *Purified water (available from chemists)*
- *Soft tissues*
- *Cotton wool balls*
- *Moisturizers from Delia Collins*
- *Water spray (e.g Evian) to refresh tired skin or fix make-up.*

MAKE-UP

Once I am satisfied that my skin is completely clean I am then ready to apply my daily make-up. To me, make-up offers an instant uplift. It allows me to highlight what is best about my face and conceal the less perfect aspects. My first experience of make-up came when I was five years old. I belonged to a dancing school when we lived in Chiswick and once took part in a show. I remember looking in the mirror and seeing these great big circles of rouge on my cheeks. Later, when I worked in the theatre, we'd slap on our 'five' and 'nine' make-up sticks for a base and hideous blue shadow on our eyes. Because we didn't have false eyelashes, we used to apply lavish black mascara and liner on our lids, extending the lines right out to the sides of our faces, almost to the same length as our eyebrows. A theatre is vast and this was done in order for the people at the back to see that we actually had eyes. We must have looked hideous. I remember one elderly actress I worked with who used to put eye black on with boiling wax. Fortunately, these days modern cosmetics are so good that I can wear the same high street brands on and off stage.

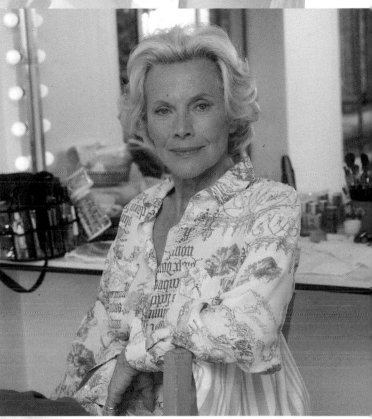

When I go out for a special evening I obviously like to look the best I can and by using my favourite products I aim to achieve a look that is both flattering and as natural as possible.

If I am spending the day at home and I'm not going to meet anyone then I think it's wonderful to have a good clean skin with nothing at all on it. However, Delia Collins always held that a woman should wear some loose powder on the skin when going out because it protects it from weather and pollution. She believed that while grit and dirt can get into the pores, loose powder sits on top of the skin protecting it. 'It has to be loose powder,' says the Delia Collins beauty expert Tina Taylor. 'Compressed powders often contain glue which can get into the pores just like dirt.'

When I'm working on *The Upper Hand* my make-up designer Sandy will make me up at the studio, but if I'm going to a function on my own then I'll do it myself, unless it is a special occasion and I'm going to be photographed in which case I'll pay a professional to do it for me.

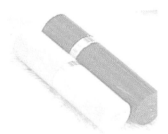

Before make-up; if you are kind to your skin and treat it considerately it will reward you.

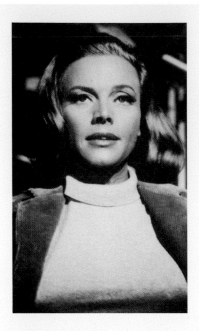

Years of professional advice has helped to shape the way I look now but it's never too late to learn new tricks.

Experiment

I'm lucky in that I can try out new looks with the help of the make-up artists on *The Upper Hand* any time I choose but if you are keen to update your look then either experiment at home or get some expert advice. Many of the make-up counters in department stores will give away free product samples if you ask or do a make-over on the spot – but be aware that they will be aiming to sell you a bag full of products into the bargain. Alternatively, you could book up to have a make-up lesson at a local beauty salon or visit one of the Green Rooms run by the Body Shop.

Tricks of the trade

One of the make-up artists I've worked with on several occasions is Jeanette Stamp and she's a great believer in de-junking your make-up bag every once in a while. 'Only carry around with you exactly what you need,' she advises. 'Leave the rest at home in a cool dark cupboard because make-up can go off. Always smell a product that you haven't used in a while and if it appears even slightly different from usual then throw it away. Liquid foundations can go rancid while mascaras shouldn't be kept for any longer than six months as anything that goes near the eye should be as clean as possible. Always buy fresh suntan lotion each year as it can go stale and consider storing perfume in the fridge as this can prolong its life for up to three years.'

Allergies

Remember that skin types can change occasionally and you may suddenly find that you are allergic to a product you've used for years.

You may also find that wearing perfume or certain pieces of jewellery in the sun may increase your skin's sensitivity.

My tip for discovering exactly what is making your skin flare up is rather drastic – it involves stopping the use of all products and gradually reintroducing them one by one over a few days. That way you should be able to discover which product is the culprit.

Remember also that acne is not something that only affects teenagers; many adults too are troubled by spots and blackheads

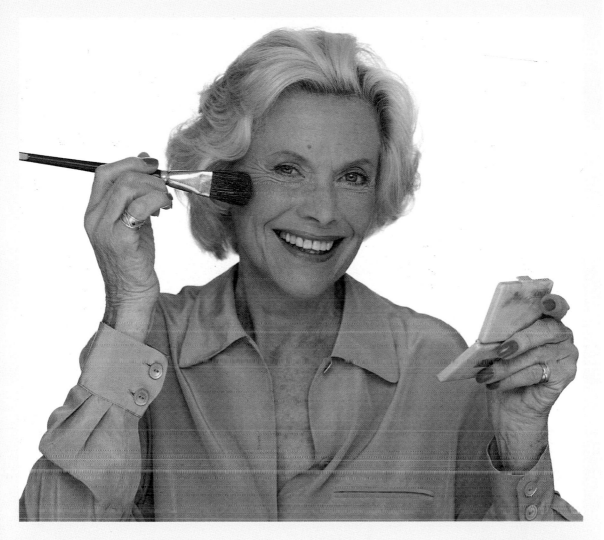

The use of good-quality brushes is a tip gained from the professionals.

that can appear at any time. If the problem is serious or upsetting don't delay in visiting your GP and getting professional help. I'm a great believer in getting problems sorted out immediately.

Evening look

Personally; I don't change my make up for day and evening looks. Even though I may be wearing richer colours in the evening, my face and hair are still the same so I tend to stick with the colours that suit me best regardless of the time of day. The only concession I make to the night is wearing more dramatic eye make-up.

TOP TIPS

When you are buying a new base, resist testing the colour on the back of your hand as it is more weathered than your face. Instead, try a little of the new product on your jawline in order to find the perfect tone (if you are wearing make-up, ask the make-up consultant to cleanse a small patch of your jaw first).

Applying make-up

I like Clinique and Estée Lauder products when I'm working and sometimes in my private life I'll apply a little of the base onto a damp sponge and gently smooth it over my skin. Experts have taught me that this is best done by starting in the middle of the face and sweeping outwards, always taking care to blend and avoid any tidemarks around the jaw or hairline – this is best achieved with the fingers.

Dark areas such as under the eyes, any deeply etched lines and the tramlines from the nose to mouth are then lightened with a little concealer on a brush and the face is then fixed with a fine dusting of translucent powder. Often I'll also use a fine spray of mineral water at this stage to help fix the look.

Alternatively, if I'm using the Delia Collins range I'll apply their colourless base and top it with a fine dusting of their loose powder which contains the necessary colour.

Blusher

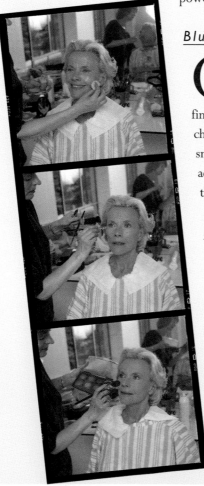

Over my cheeks I'll lightly brush a very natural sweep of soft, sandy pink blusher. I find the best way to do this is to find the cheekbone with my fingers and then simply sweep the brush under the bone from cheek to temple. Alternatively, I'll do a little Mona Lisa smile and brush along under the cheek. The effect I aim to achieve is a blended, healthy glow – there's nothing worse than a stripe of harsh colour or false, round rosy cheeks.

Eyes

I've found that the colours which suit my eyes best are smoky greys and soft browns. A couple of years ago there was a fashion for hot colours like oranges and smudgy browns and on *The Upper Hand* we went with the fashion but they really didn't suit me at all – they seemed to make my eyes pop out. My eyes are a soft blue so I allow my natural colour to dominate and not the eye shadow. I've found that flatter, matt tones suit my skin best – anything that is pearlized or contains too much sparkle tends to pick up the lines in older skin and emphasize them.

Eye shadow

Eye shadow should be applied to the deepest part of the socket, not the lid, for maximum effect. Sometimes using a combination of too many colours only has the effect of closing in the eyes and making them look smaller. I aim for the most natural finish every time, with pale eyelids and soft brown sockets widening towards the outer edge of the lid.

I've also learnt that eye liner opens the eyes out. You don't have to end up looking like Cleopatra in order to get some definition and you should aim to achieve a smudged effect on the bottom lid and finer line on the top. If you've never used eye liner before then practise a few times before putting it on for a special occasion. Eye liner needs a steady hand and whether you're using a liquid or pencil you should work from the centre of the eye outwards. I've always found that a block and brush works best for me.

If you make a mistake then use use a damp cotton bud dipped in some fresh water. Never be tempted to spit in a block liner as you could easily pass on an infection from a cold sore in this way.

It's always a good idea to practise any new make-up technique before a special occasion. I remember once deciding to try false eyelashes on the night of a glizty film première in the Fifties. I got into such a state with them that I ended up glueing my eyes open. When I shook hands with Prince Philip he gave me a very odd look because I quite simply couldn't close my eyes. He must have wondered why I looked permanently astonished.

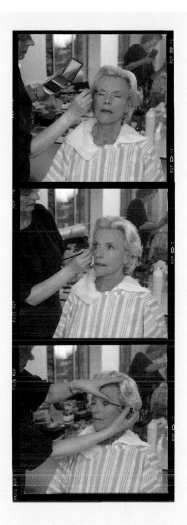

Mascara

Mascara is vital for me because I am a natural blonde and my eyelashes are not very dark. I always use an eyelash curler first, followed by a lash primer (Estée Lauder do an excellent one which is white) followed by two coats of mascara using a long, straight brush. I hate clogging, so I'll always use an eyelash comb next. Some women make the mistake of loading the mascara wand too heavily by frantically dipping it into the container. If there is too much mascara on the brush, wipe it with a tissue and then use it.

I always use brushes to apply any form of eye make-up and take great pains to keep them scrupulously clean.

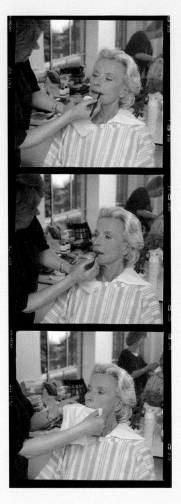

TOP LIP TIPS

- The secret of permanent colour is to keep blotting when you're applying lipstick. Kiss a folded tissue between coats and your colour should last all day.

- Use a powder puff or brush loaded with a little powder to gently buff and seal the edges just before the final coat of lipstick goes on.

- When choosing a new lipstick try testing the colour on the pad of your index finger, rather than on the back of your hand – you'll find that the colour is more suited to your natural lip colour there.

- If you're planning to buy new colours for the spring or summer, look out for lipsticks containing an SPF (Sun Protection Factor) as lips are particularly vulnerable to sun damage.

- In America you can buy a product called Carmex which is brilliant for 'fixing' lipstick and is also excellent for chapped or dry lips. In Britain, try Elizabeth Arden's Lipfix.

Lips

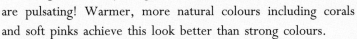

I absolutely hate bright red lipsticks and make-up artists are always trying to put them on me. I find very bright lipsticks unattractive. Make-up is supposed to highlight what is good about you. I think the best kind of lipstick should make you look healthy and rosy – you know, like when your lips are throbbing and even your gums are pulsating! Warmer, more natural colours including corals and soft pinks achieve this look better than strong colours.

One brilliant discovery I've made lately is wax lip liner. Body Shop do an excellent one called No Wander and as the name suggests it prevents the lip gloss or lipstick from bleeding out.

When applying any kind of lip liner try to keep the wrist relaxed and the movement fluid. Work from the outside inwards in order to get a smooth line and if you make a mistake correct with a cotton bud.

When I'm doing it all properly, I'll just apply Elizabeth Arden's lip fix, then a colourless wax pencil, followed by lip pencil, a smudge of Eight Hour Cream from Elizabeth Arden and a soft brown lip base, and lastly a soft pink applied with a lip brush.

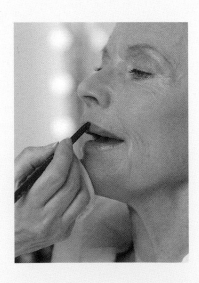

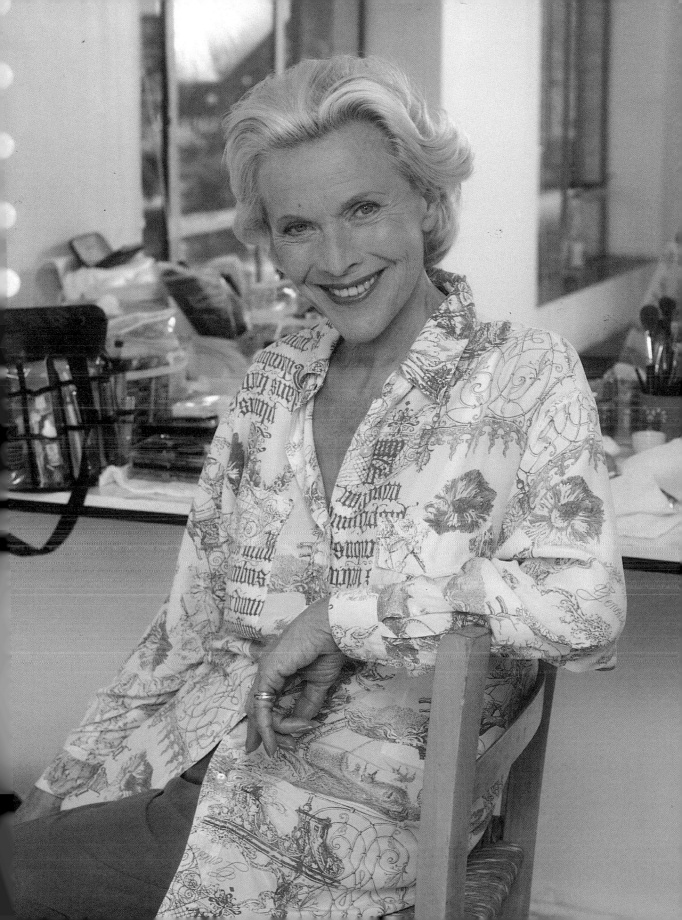

TANNING

I love to tan and I must admit that over the years I've abused my skin dreadfully by lying out in the sun for too long and using sun oils with little or no protection factor in them. My only defence is that I didn't know about the dangers of skin cancer then – but I certainly do now. If I get too much sun I get herpes on my lips.

I've been lucky enough to enjoy holidays in the most exotic parts of the world from Barbados to Fiji but these days I wouldn't dream of sitting out in the sun without a floppy hat, sunglasses and a selection of sun creams. I find the best way to tan safely is to build up gradually. I like to accustom my skin to the sun slowly by using a lotion that contains a high SPF (sun protection factor) for the first few days and only staying in the sun for a short while during the cooler times of the day.

I always apply my lotion generously before going into the sun and slap on more every two hours and after swimming. Through experience I've learnt that it's also possible to burn on cloudy days and it's not a good idea to underestimate the strength of British sun, either.

According to the Cancer Research Campaign we should all avoid the sun between 11am and 3pm, wear loose clothing when we walk about and seek natural shade in the form of trees or other shelter where possible. When choosing your correct SPF you need to work out how long you can naturally stay in the sun without burning. If, for example, it's 10 minutes and you choose a SPF10, you will be able to stay safely in the sun for 10 × 10 minutes, or about an hour and 40 minutes. Always read the label on the sun lotion carefully and don't skimp on sunblock for sensitive areas like tips of the ears, nose or lips. Afterwards, remoisturizing is essential.

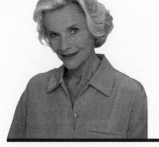

'I feel instantly uplifted when I've got a tan, but these days I'm very careful when it comes to sunbathing.'

Faking it

Skin experts say the most intelligent way to tan these days is to fake it and there is now a huge variety of really good fake tans being sold by everyone from Clarins to the Body Shop.

Self-tanning creams work by reacting with the proteins in the skin and can give you a healthy glow within hours. If you want to achieve the best results, it doesn't pay to rush the process. Dedicate an evening to yourself and get it right.

- *Firstly, shower down and get the body scrupulously clean.*
- *Moisturize with your favourite light body lotion.*
- *Wait half an hour and then smooth on a thin, even layer of self-tan. Take care over darker areas like the elbows and ankles to ensure that the coverage is equal.*
- *Add more layers for a deeper tan and always wash your hands afterwards unless you find orange hands attractive.*
- *Take time for the lotion to dry onto the skin. Wait at least half an hour before going to bed or getting dressed to prevent colour rubbing off on sheets or clothes.*

Remember that you should never use self-tan instead of a sun protection cream. Allow your self-tan to develop overnight and apply a SPF before you go in the sun again.

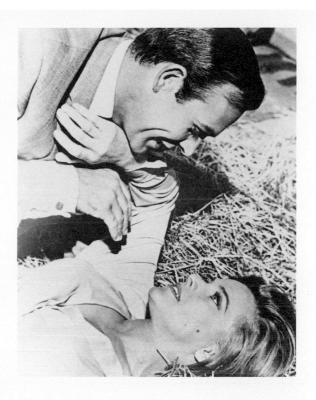

On medical advice, I had my famous black mole removed. It was a shame but it had to be done.

Warning signs

Each year there are now 28,000 new cases of skin cancer and over 1,500 deaths. The leg is the most common place for a woman to find a cancer, usually between the ankle and knee, but if the spot is found early enough there's usually a 90 per cent chance of recovery.

According to the Department of Health, we should all look out for moles which are:

- *Getting larger*
- *Have an irregular outline or are different colours of brown and black*
- *Are bigger than the blunt end of a pencil*
- *Itch, bleed or are sore.*

If you look back at old pictures you will see that I used to have a mole on my cheek. I have had it removed because it was getting blacker and blacker.I miss it.

NAILS

Some people might regard having a manicure as something of an indulgence but for me it's a necessity. I have only had professional manicures in the last few years, but as I'm absolutely hopeless at doing my nails myself I must say that a really good manicure or pedicure is a wonderful treat. I like my nails to look well manicured and I'm perfectly sure my character Laura West in *The Upper Hand* would insist upon it. Some women spend hours on their make-up and leave their hands looking like a fright. Unlike the face, hands have few natural oils and for anyone who regularly gets their hands wet through washing up or looking after children, moisture needs to be replaced daily.

One of the best hand creams I've found is Vaseline's Intensive Care lotion, which is non-greasy and affordable, while for luxury I like Clarins hand cream. After a hideous experience in Spain once when a manicurist hacked at my cuticles with scissors, I now only allow my cuticles to be clipped if absolutely necessary, as they soon become hard if you cut them. Nails are best kept smart by filing them (in one direction) with one of those black emery boards (I never use scissors). There's nothing worse than chipped nail varnish, so unless I can make an invisible running repair I always take my varnish off as soon as it begins to flake.

Gloves

I try to wear gloves in the winter, as they are protective and elegant too. While at home the same applies with rubber gloves when I'm doing any cleaning or washing around my home. When I remember, I actually put on two pairs, cotton ones first and rubber ones on top (because I can't bear that awful smelly dampness when you take off rubber gloves) Often, however, I find myself launching into a task and before I know it I'm wrist-deep in the hoover bag with nothing protective on my hands at all, which I instantly regret.

FEET

Years of wearing fashionable shoes have left most women's feet in a dreadful state and I have to admit that mine are no more beautiful than anybody else's.

It's a misconception that we keep the same shoe size for life.

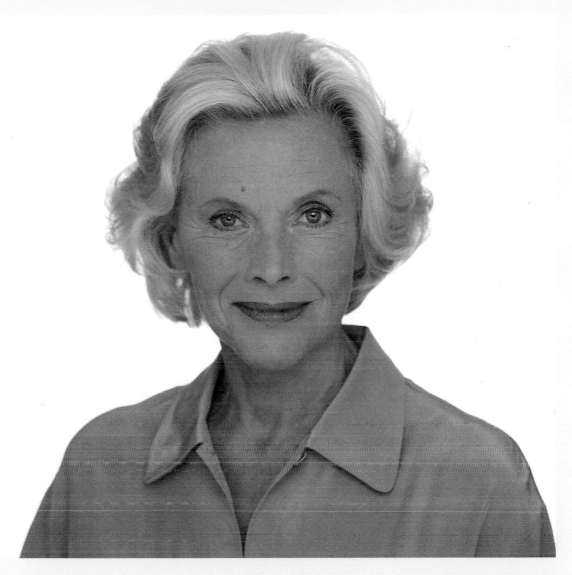

The size of our feet can change, especially after childbirth, so bear that in mind the next time you buy a pair of shoes if you've recently put on weight.

Swollen joints and corns are common, and only regular visits to a chiropodist can sort these problems out. On a daily basis, however, there is still plenty we can do. Feet should be washed and carefully dried every day, with hard skin being removed with a pumice stone as often as possible. A moisturizing cream like Body Shop's famous Peppermint Foot Cream can be applied and the nails should be clipped straight across to avoid in-growing.

I like my everyday make-up to be flattering yet subtle.

TEETH

Sparkling teeth radiate good health and I take particular care of mine. According to dentists, on the whole we're now keeping our teeth for longer which is just as it should be, considering a healthy tooth should outlast its owner.

Now that we understand how destructive sugar is to our teeth we're having less fillings, but plaque and gum disease continue to plague us. Only by regular cleaning, flossing and trips to the hygienist can these problems be kept in check.

There is no point in brushing from side to side – that won't shift food particles or acid lodged between the teeth. It's vital to brush from top to bottom on the top jaw and bottom to top on the lower jaw. Dentists recommend you brush for at least three minutes a day, twice a day, especially after a meal. According to the British Dental Association, a toothbrush should have nylon filaments with round ends and be no harder than medium texture; the head size should be no bigger than one and a half back teeth, and you should change your toothbrush every two months instead of the national average of every 10 months. As one grows older slight gaps do tend to appear between the teeth, so I also favour a dental 'bottle' brush (it looks just like a miniature version of the kind of brush you'd clean a baby's bottle with), which I find cleans my teeth well.

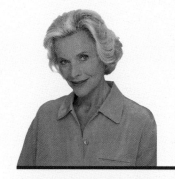

*'I'm not as fanatical about my teeth as is Laura in **The Upper Hand**, but I do care about them.'*

HAIR

Until about 12 years ago my hair was naturally blonde but instead of going grey it started going dark. Now it has assistance to stay blonde. I have a lot of it, it is very fine and it's a b****r to manage myself! I absolutely adore having my hair brushed, and I think one of the most perfect beauty treatments I've ever had was in Singapore. I had my hair washed and they gave me a wonderful head massage as part of it. It was a dreamy, dreamy experience. They used their nails and it was half massage and half scratch. Heaven.

My hairstyle has become something of a trademark and I've pretty much kept the same swept-back style, off my face, look

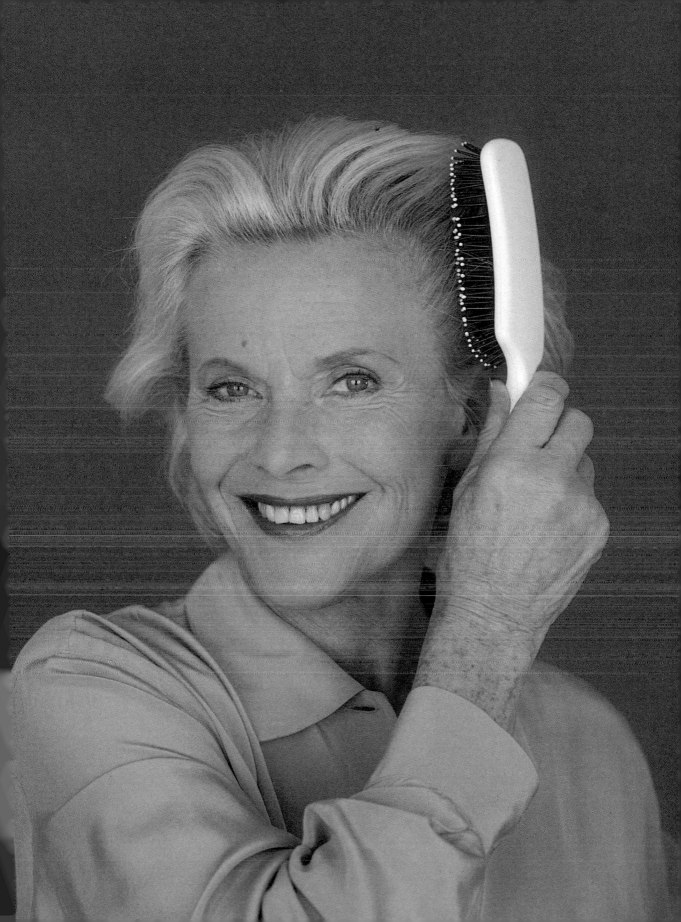

TOP TIPS

* Remember that when your hair is wet it loses much of its elasticity, so excessive combing may make it break. The best discoveries I've made recently are spray-in conditioners and serum sprays. The conditioners are perfect for fine hair like mine as they allow me to instantly detangle and protect my hair without incurring static, while serum sprays help strengthen weak or brittle hair and make it shine.

* Once in a while, and especially after a holiday in the sun, I'll give my hair a real treat and invest in a tub of hair wax or a cream mask. After shampooing I massage the treatment wax into my hair, wrap a warm towel around it and leave it on for at least 20 minutes. I then give it another quick shampoo and allow my hair to dry naturally. The result is silky, shiny hair.

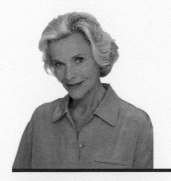

'My hair has been the bane of my life. There's lots of it but it's got a mind of its own.'

since my Avengers days. I have found that it's a style that suited my face then and still flatters me now. I did have a fringe once but I spent the whole time shoving it out of my eyes so that didn't last long. I've been going to the same hairdresser in Central London for several years and honestly believe that a good haircut is something worth investing in.

You may pay a fortune for clothes which you only wear once in a while but your hair is on show every day, so why not have it looking the best it can? My hair rolls up in curlers easily but the curls fall out just as quickly in damp weather. When I was younger every director adored my hair before shooting but once we were launched into a scene he'd cry 'Cut! Do something about that goddam hair!' because it was obscuring my face.

Hair care

Just as with my skin, I treat my hair very kindly. Our hair reflects our state of health and as hair is a living thing that sheds and replaces itself daily, if we don't take care of it it will soon look dull and lifeless. It's estimated that we start to lose our hair at around 30, but there is plenty we can do to keep it looking good for many years after that. The biggest enemy of hair is overdrying. When I wash my hair at home I try not to overuse a heated brush or rollers. Instead I let my hair dry naturally for as long as possible and use them at the end. Whenever I use my hairdryer I never switch it to the hot setting. Heated rollers, tongs and high-powered dryers may help to tease your hair into shape but they remove essential oils at the same time. Harsh perms and colour treatments will play havoc too. I find that regularly changing the brand of my shampoo and conditioner helps to stop my hair getting used to certain products.

Before washing I give my hair a good combing to loosen any dirt and to untangle it. If I wash my hair in the bath, I use the shower after the first dunking as it is vital to cleanse it with fresh, clean water.

To wash it I simply wet the hair with warm water and apply a little shampoo to my fingertips. Then, starting at the forehead, I massage the shampoo into the hair in small circular movements. 'Doesn't everybody?' you'll say, but the aim is to clean the hair AND improve circulation.

Once the hair is squeaky clean, and this may take two washes if my hair is full of hair spray after a show, I apply a generous blob of creamy conditioner to the ends, comb it through and then wait for about five minutes before rinsing again.

COSMETIC SURGERY

Although I'm a strong advocate of the importance of natural beauty, I'm lucky. I have good hair, good skin and a body that responds well to exercise but that's not to say that I wouldn't consider cosmetic surgery if I thought it was necessary. One of the best non-surgical little products I've come across are called Frownies*. These small, self adhesive pieces of brown paper are applied to the frown lines and wrinkles between your eyes at night and work by holding the underlying facial muscles firmly in place. Apparently this allows the muscles time to regain their strength and tone and the result is a smoother skin.

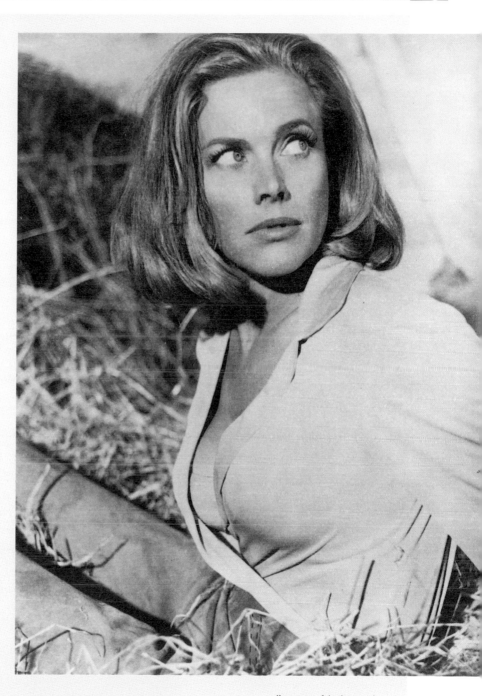

I've never felt the need for breast implants – I think you can see why. Having a large bust has been a mixed blessing.

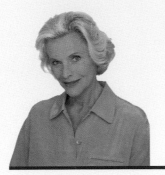

'Everyone has something which is beautiful about them, whether it's a lovely smile or a bubbling personality. But if you feel the need to have cosmetic surgery, then that's your choice.'

I doubt though if I would ever have a full face lift, it's not something that appeals to me. Besides, face lifts need to be done early on in life and regularly if one is not to fall to pieces in between each op. I'm not a great fan of treatments like liposuction (whereby fat is sucked out of overweight areas), either. I'd much prefer that women should have sufficient discipline over their diet not to get to such a stage. It's what we eat that shapes how we look. Diet and exercise are the only way to remove fat and restore shape permanently.

Breast implants, however, are another matter. I've always had a large bosom which has had its advantages and disadvantages. I remember once going to see an acupuncturist while I was touring with a play which was very emotional, giving me frequent headaches. As I came out from behind the screen with just my knickers on as requested he took one look at me and said, 'Christ, woman, what a pair of tits.' Very professional! For women who are tempted to have breast implants then I say, why not?

It's usually best to wait until your childbearing days are over before having implants. Although you can still breastfeed with implants, problems tend to arise after breastfeeding stops. Because the breast skin has stretched so much, once for the silicone implants and again for the milk, many women find that their breasts have drooped down to their knees and they need to have a second, expensive fix-up operation to stop the descent. If you wait until all the kids are out of the way then you'll only have to have one operation, and as there's always an element of risk involved in having a general anaesthetic, that has got to be preferable to two.

My only advice to anyone considering cosmetic surgery is to get the best possible treatment. Go first to your family doctor and get a referral rather than respond to newspaper ads. Save up, go to the best in the business and before you commit yourself ask if you may speak to some of the other patients he or she has already treated.

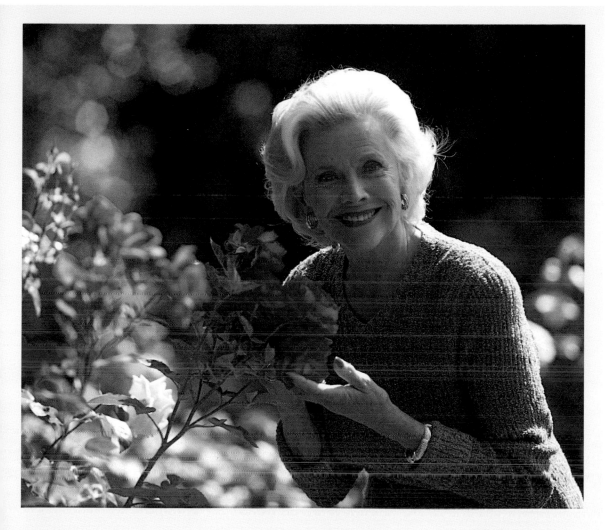

ENJOY

There was a song that we used to sing when we were children on holiday in Littlehampton called 'Keep Young And Beautiful'. That was the first line, and the second line went 'It's your duty to be beautiful'. I firmly believe that we have a duty to ourselves – not to anyone else – to maintain our looks. If you know that you look your absolute best it will affect every aspect of your life and with that will come the confidence to keep moving forwards and to enjoy life to the full.

Make the most of every new day . Be positive about life and enjoy the moment.

* Frownies are available by mail order from:
Cassina France, 28 Cavendish Road, London, E4 9NH.

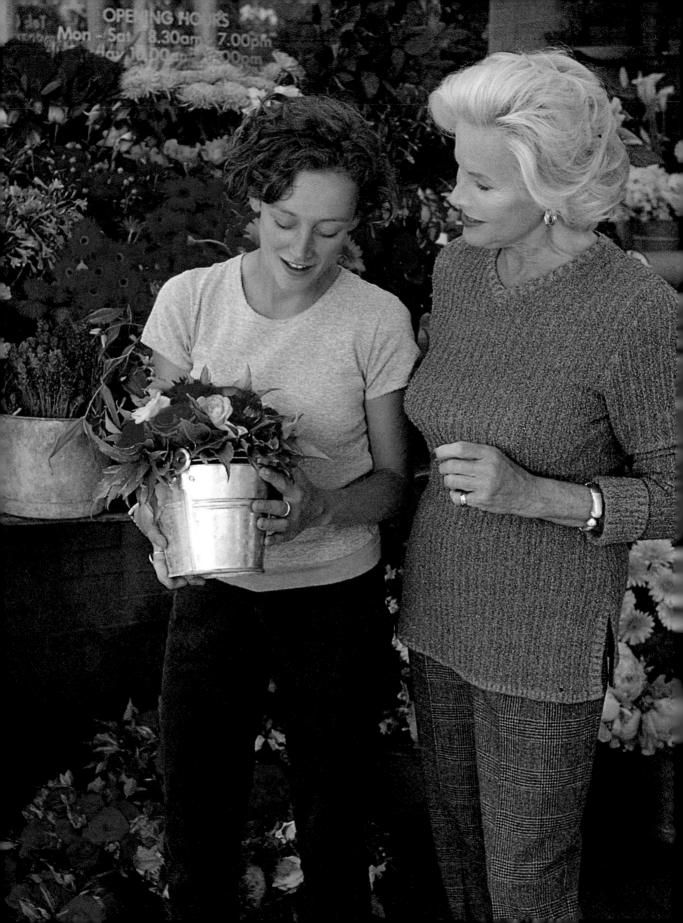

TRY A LITTLE PAMPERING

There's nothing like some tender loving care to help revitalize the body and restore the spirit. I find I respond terribly well to a little pampering. It can be something as simple as a new bar of exquisitely scented soap or a wonderfully fragrant dish of pot pourri, but as long as my treat is something that appeals to my senses and lifts my mood I feel instantly revived. I love some of the totally unnecessary things in life with a passion: beautifully perfumed oils for the bath, Belgian chocolates or even smoked salmon through the post as a surprise. My idea of luxury is curling up in a soft dressing gown eating a delicious chocolate after a soothing, fragrant bath. When we were children growing up in West London, the whole family, six of us, shared one bathroom and one towel. I don't know how often it was changed but I suspect it was weekly. When we had our bath on a Friday night we would all splash about in the water and then attempt to dry off with the one towel in the house – it was dried briefly on the fireguard, but bad luck if you were last. Consequently I now consider a bath towel to be the most luxurious item in the world. To me a thick, all-encompassing bath sheet is luxury beyond belief.

I like things to look, feel and smell just right. Flowers make me feel indulged too and I enjoy sending and receiving them. As I don't have a garden I especially like planted bowls of flowers which continue to grow in the house. I'm hopeless at arranging flowers but I love it when people give them to me, particularly when they are brilliantly put together in a bunch and all I have to do is put them in a vase of water.

CONTENTS

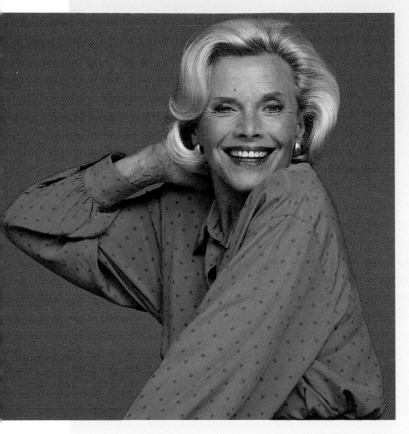

I have always believed that true beauty comes from within.

Since I've been doing my own show I've kept all the silk ribbons which come wrapped around bouquets, which I still think are wonderfully glamorous, and have used them to decorate a little table in the hall of my apartment. When I first started receiving flowers at the beginning of my career I felt extremely special and that thrill has never faded. In August 1996, when I celebrated my seventieth birthday, my home was filled with flowers and I was intoxicated with their scent. My favourite flowers are white spider chrysanthemums and, of course, I love roses. I am not potty about orchids and I won't have anemones in the house. Although carnations are pretty, I really prefer pinks because their perfume is so lovely. Scent is terribly important to me. I really dislike cooking smells lingering after the meal is over, particularly that of fish. The kitchen window is flung open and Floris fragrance is sprayed here there and everywhere.

I almost always wear perfume myself – I don't really feel finished without it. During the daytime I like Yves St. Laurent's Paris and in the evening I'll wear Femme by Rochas – those are two firm favourites. Yves St. Laurent's Y had a long run, as did Estée Lauder's White Linen, and I may go back to them. I do like to vary what I use otherwise it becomes boring. In the bath I like to use Femme again.

Friends are always giving me pot pourri and scented candles as gifts, which I love. I like my home to smell fresh, as there is something invigorating about smelling good and living in delicious surroundings. I firmly believe that a little pampering has a very proper place in our whole well-being. It's isn't selfish or vain to take care of ourselves, to pay attention to the whole body or to treat it kindly with relaxing treatments. I would rather have a massage than an anti-depressant pill from the doctor any time.

If a pampering treatment makes you feel good about yourself then you couldn't do yourself a greater favour. To me, pampering equates health and a calmness of mind. I believe in self-help and preventative medicine and you could say that I give my body constant care with the healthy foods I feed it and the extra help I give it by way of exercise and relaxing treatments. I enjoy reflexology and massage, which allow me to feel good about myself and contribute to my general well-being too.

TOP TO TOE – HOME TREATMENTS

One of the biggest treats I've enjoyed in recent years is visiting health spas. For sheer hedonistic pampering they can't be beaten. No longer the elitist institutions they once were, health spas are now dotted all around the country and people from all walks of life go to them. If you can't afford to go to one for a week or weekend, get a friend to buy you a day pass to one as a birthday treat and enjoy several hours of undisturbed bliss away from the pressures of everyday life. I find such places absolutely perfect for study. It is bliss to have a massage after breakfast, learn until lunch and then have some pampering treatment which allows one to digest what one has learnt before returning to learning physically relaxed. It is not the management's idea of the best use of their facilities, however, as the emphasis is on total relaxation.

If visiting a health spa is not possible, there is nothing to stop you from creating your own beauty sanctuary at home.

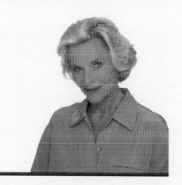

Plan well in advance and choose a weekend when you know you'll be able to farm the children out to willing friends or relatives. Persuade your man to go off with the chaps (now that shouldn't be hard) and simply devote some time to yourself. One of the secrets of really looking and feeling half your age for the rest of your life is taking some time out to be by yourself and do something just for YOU once in a while.

'Take the time to indulge yourself thoroughly once in a while – your blood pressure will thank you for it!'

* *Before you start, stop by at the supermarket and stock up with lots of healthy salads, fresh foods, fruits and juices.*

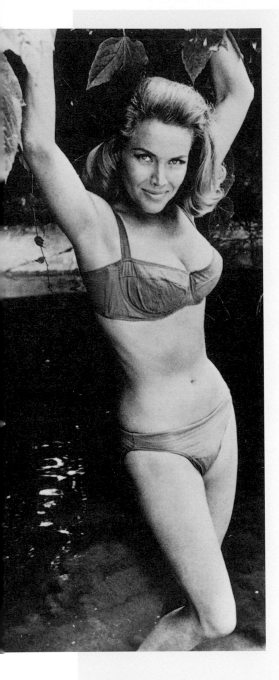

Whoops. . .

- *Buy foods that will be easy to prepare for the next couple of days.*
- *Give away or throw away any junk foods, biscuits or chocolates you may be tempted by.*
- *Ban yourself from having tea and coffee and give your body the chance to restore itself.*
- *Warm a huge bundle of soft towels in the airing cupboard — you're going to need them.*
- *Tell your friends what you are planning to do.*
- *Unplug the phone.*
- *Put some atmospheric music on the cassette or CD player.*

Friday night

The best way to slough away the old you is to plunge into a luxurious bubble bath. I love to fill my bathroom with fragrant pot pourri, fresh flowers and even scented candles when I want to pamper myself and feel as if I'm wafting off on a cloud.

- *Once you are clean all over, rub a little sea salt on your elbows to remove any dead skin — I am fiercely against harsh scrubs or exfoliators of any kind either for the face or body.*
- *Over your super-smooth skin, now massage in lashings of rich body lotion and wrap yourself in a huge, warm, soft towel. Put a couple of pieces of sliced cucumber over your eyes and take at least 15 minutes in which to just relax.*
- *Apply your usual night cream and retire to bed for an early night. Going to bed well before midnight often gives me the best night's sleep of all.*

Saturday

Throughout the whole weekend, ensure that you keep drinking plenty of water. My daughter gave me a water purifier and I drink 1.2 litres (2pt/5 cups) a day; half before breakfast and the rest during the day, finishing at about 4pm as I'm not keen on going to the bathroom all night long! I've found that it cleanses my system and makes me feel fresh and alert.

- *Now that your body is clean and smooth, dedicate some time to your face. I go for regular facials and again these are very gentle. Firstly, cleanse your face in your usual way and then gently steam it. Add* some fresh, chopped herbs to boiled water in a bowl to make it smell nice. Put a towel over your head and place your face above the bowl for as long as the water is still steaming. Take care not to get too close to the water or burn the skin. Repeat three times and then splash the face with cool water or wipe it with purified water on cotton wool, as I do.

- Now select a nourishing face pack to apply. Don't opt for one that will dry and harden on your face — instead, choose a creamy mask that will remoisturize and replenish. If you don't have a favourite product you can always whip up one yourself.

- The only beauty tip that my mother ever gave me was that whipped-up egg whites are good for the skin. So they are, if your skin is young and prone to being oily. Citrus fruits will also work well on young skin to make it less greasy. Mashed peach is good for irritated skin, while melon slices make good compresses for tired eyes. If your skin is drier, use an egg yolk or a mashed-up avocado or banana on your face to help remoisturize it. Simply mash up half an avocado or a banana with a spoonful of honey, whizz around in the blender, lie down flat and apply. Leave on for about 10 minutes for maximum cleansing then rinse off with warm water. Experiment with what you've got in the fridge and make up your own combinations — for once you've got the time!

- With a beautifully clean face you can now pluck your eyebrows if you wish. Always pluck from underneath the brow, following its natural line, and never pull the hair back against the follicle. Remove rogue hairs from the upper lip and chin with sterilized tweezers.

- Now go for a long walk. Dress in loose, comfortable clothes and good walking shoes or trainers and take the time to really stride out and get some fresh air in those lungs. At a health spa you'd no doubt be attending exercise classes as well as having beauty treatments, so don't stint on the exertion just because you are at home.

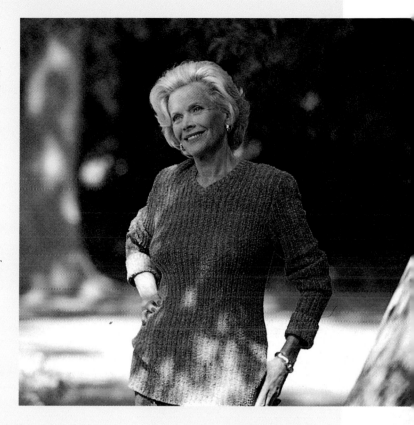

I've always been a fresh-air fiend. I thrive on being out and about.

Sunday

Make the most of this day by yourself to really calm the mind. So many of us have frantic days in our lives but rarely balance them with totally relaxing ones. Don't forget that your body and mind sometimes need time just to rest and that's not something that you should ever feel guilty about.

- *Get up early and go for a swim — that way you should get to the local pool well ahead of the family groups. Try to do at least 10 lengths of the pool or 12 minutes of nonstop swimming in order to increase your metabolic rate. Many leisure centres now have sauna and steam rooms, but I steer well clear of them as I am not keen on intense heat. Instead, shower down using a refreshing shower gel, wash and condition your hair. Towel dry it and allow it to dry naturally. If it is not warm enough outside then dry it with a hairdryer before you leave. I've found that moisturizers are the key to supple, young-looking skin, so I always ensure that my skin never dries out and is constantly replenished. Moisturise your entire body after swimming.*

- *Try giving your feet a real treat by investing in a jar of good old Vaseline. Soak them in some warm soapy water and while they are still damp, massage in some foot scrub (Crabtree & Evelyn do a good one). Wrap your feet in clingfilm and relax for about 10 minutes. Next, rinse and gently dry the feet, then liberally apply Vaseline all over them and pop on a pair of cotton socks. (For maximum effect, you could even wear the socks to bed and your feet will feel wonderfully soft and smooth in the morning.)*

- *Finish off by applying a couple of coats of your favourite nail colour. Apply a base coat from the bottom to the tip of each toe, working from the big toe to the small one. Then add two coats of your favourite colour on top, allowing at least five minutes in between each coat for the colour to dry properly.*

- *Hands can be made baby soft by dipping them in paraffin wax which has been boiled and allowed to cool. Leave the cooled wax on for 30 minutes. Next give yourself a home manicure. Start by removing all traces of old nail varnish with some acetone-free remover. Next soak the nails in a bowl of warm soapy water and then gently massage in some cuticle cream. Rinse again and dry*

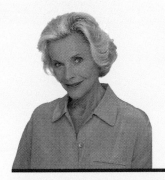

'We should never feel guilty about relaxing occasionally. The body needs a period of rest from time to time.'

thoroughly. Use a wooden emery board —
the black ones are best, as the grit is less
harsh. Shape the nails by using large,
sweeping strokes in one direction each time
— never be tempted to 'saw' your nails.

- When they are ready to paint, apply a
  base coat to each nail and allow to dry
  for at least four minutes. Always wipe the
  brush against the far side of the pot.
  Apply two coats of your chosen varnish,
  allowing five minutes between each coat
  and then a final layer of top coat.

- Fix the colour either by spraying on a nail
  fixing product or plunging the nails into
  a bowl of iced water. Allow the nails as
  long as possible to dry before you do
  anything else.

- For a really professional effect, it's now
  possible to buy French Polish manicure kits
  which include the base coat and varnish
  in shades of pink and in white to give a
  really chic finish.

- Use the afternoon to unwind completely.
  Read a favourite book or listen to the kind
  of music you love the most. If nothing else, just sit quietly and
  think. I find that meditation is extremely calming and can help
  reduce stress.

- Like many actors, I enjoy the benefits of aromatherapy massage. I
  find that a soothing massage using specially blended aromatherapy
  oils is the perfect way for me to relieve stress and relax both the
  mind and muscles. Not everyone can afford to have an
  aromatherapist come to their home, so it's helpful that several
  companies like Neal's Yard and Tisserand sell products which
  already have aromatherapy oils in them. Invest in something like
  Tisserand's Relaxing Body Lotion which contains the warm properties
  of orange blossom, bergamot and lavender blended with aloe vera.
  Gently massage the lotion all over your skin and retire to bed.

- By Monday morning you'll be looking like a dream and feeling like
  a superstar — and you'll have done it all for the cost of a few products.

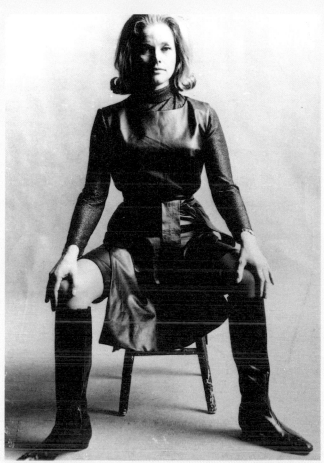

Cathy Gale didn't worry
about her nails — they
were short and
functional. I like mine to
be glamorous.

MASSAGE

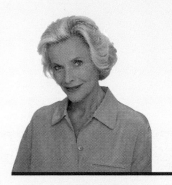

Massage is one of the treatments I allow myself on a regular basis. There is nothing more relaxing than the wonderful sensation of a qualified masseuse (in my case) gently kneading and stroking the muscles of my body. I find the pure sensation of touch to be most beneficial to my mental and physical state. Ideally I would like to have a massage every other week, but realistically it usually works out at once a month. Jill Wootton, my masseuse, usually spends about an hour and a half on me and combines reflexology, massage and aromatherapy. 'I start by placing my hands on the feet,' she explains. 'This aids general relaxation and allows me to find out what is going on in the rest of the body. I can pick up energy levels and "tune in" to problems that way.'

'If I could afford to have only one pampering treatment I think it would have to be massage.'

The kind of massage I prefer involves rhythmical, fluid movements and I would run a mile from anyone who tried to 'chop' or slap my skin. 'I don't think I've done a Swedish massage since the day I qualified,' says Jill. 'People who need to relax and reduce stress benefit much more from a gentler form of massage.'

Not only is a massage relaxing but it can relieve muscle tension caused by stress, increase blood flow and make the skin more supple. It is also thought that massage may release endorphins, morphine-like substances which are nature's most powerful painkillers. Aromatherapy is a form of massage which involves the use of essential oils (pure aromatic plant oils) and Jill also incorporates the use of these in my treatment. They restore well-being by stimulating the body's own natural healing process. Essential oils don't only smell delicious, they can actively treat conditions such as migraine, high blood pressure and insomnia. Because they are so potent, such oils should only be used with care — for example basil, fennel and sage are just three oils which should be avoided at all costs during pregnancy.

For me, Jill will select the appropriate oil to match my needs on that particular day. If I am staying in and want to be calm she'll use an oil like vetivert which is very grounding, but if I am going out or planning to work that night she'll use lemon, which is lighter and less sedating. Essential oils all do different things: lavender aids sleep, geranium lifts the spirits, while camomile is a wonderful soother.

When I have a massage I ensure that the room is warm and slightly darkened. I unplug the phone and fax and ignore the door bell as I prepare for my time of sheer pleasure. A good masseuse should always take a detailed account of your medical history before starting and will suggest you see a doctor if she finds something unusual during the treatment. There are also times when you shouldn't have a massage, including when you have a high temperature, a skin infection or any kind of infectious disease, or if you're suffering from an inflammatory condition like thrombosis. Massage can be expensive but I think that it is money well spent. It depends on where your priorities lie – you'd probably spend the same amount going out for a meal once a month. My masseuse is freelance so I'm lucky in that she is able to come to my home and treat me in the comfort of my own surroundings.

But massage doesn't always have to be done by a professional giving your partner a slow, lingering massage is the perfect way of bringing the two of you closer together. Use a carrier oil like sweet almond, or even baby or vegetable oil. Choose a time when you won't be disturbed, light a scented candle and get him to lie on a towel on the bed. Put a little oil onto one palm and gently warm it by rubbing both hands together. Start with light movements, massaging your hands gently but firmly across the skin. Make the movements fluid and broad and avoid breaking contact. Begin at the back of the neck where tension builds up and gradually work your hands down the body as gently or firmly as you both feel happy with. Just do what feels right for the two of you – who knows what it may lead to! I find my massages help relieve stress and soothe my muscles, but more than that they make me feel wonderfully indulged and smelling heavenly.

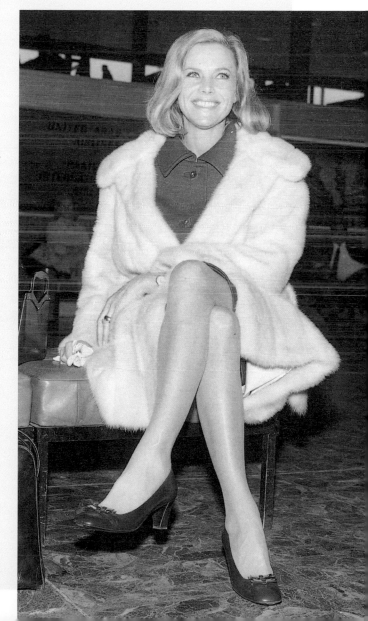

Me in my luxurious palomino mink coat, long ago sold

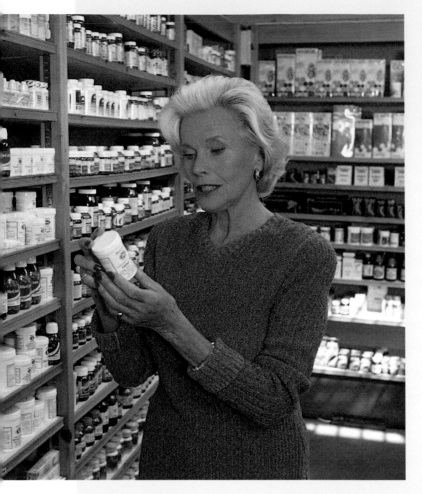

I'm interested in all forms of alternative medicine and keep a completely open mind.

REFLEXOLOGY

Some people hate having their feet touched, but I love it. The practice of reflexology is as ancient as the Egyptian pyramids and as indulgent as any beauty treatment. I was introduced to it by a woman called Ellen Sunde in Brighton. I have reflexology at home but it is much, much more than simple foot massage. Reflexology doesn't tickle or hurt – the reflexologist gently but firmly uses her fingers and thumbs to apply pressure to various parts of the foot. The belief is that certain points on the foot correspond to other parts of your body – the foot is a map of your body, if you like. Therefore, if gentle pressure is applied to particular parts of the feet, energy will begin to follow and this will act on problem areas and help the body to overcome the ailment. Massaging specific points works to stimulate blood circulation and the lymphatic system, which results in increasing energy levels and elimination of toxins. Done properly, reflexology can help cure any number of ailments from bulimia to backache (which is perfect for me), plus migraine, irritable bowel syndrome and asthma. It has also been found to be helpful in the treatment of cancer patients because while it doesn't cure the cancer it can go some way towards stimulating the body and helping the immune system to function better.

When I'm having reflexology I feel as though all my energy channels are being unblocked. I feel wonderfully relaxed and all tension goes.

OSTEOPATHY

Thumping my spine as I did regularly in *The Avengers* has not helped my back. Therefore as well as concentrating on my Pilates classes, where correct balance and posture are encouraged, I also visit an osteopath. My osteopath has a light touch and manipulates my back into shape again with the minimum of dramatics, his finger pressure relaxing my muscles. I only go when I need to and that's usually when I've carried five bags of heavy shopping! One side of my back is worse than the other and when it goes my spine actually bows outwards at waist level. My osteopath believes that because many of us have sedentary jobs which involve sitting down all day, we don't stretch out our muscles enough. One movement he's shown me, therefore, is to stand on one leg and pull the heel of the other foot up to my bottom. I try to do this every day and it really does seem to help my posture. I try to be aware of the dangers to my back in everyday life: I bend my knees when I lift anything heavy, try to avoid stooping over the washing-up and take frequent breaks when I'm driving long distances, but like everyone else I am not infallible and there is always that unguarded moment.

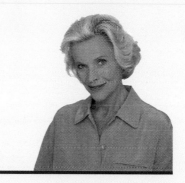

'Stress is causing more illnesses than ever before. It's something I take great pains to keep under control.'

I'm delighted that these days there is more of a crossover between traditional and alternative methods of treating conditions. Some hospitals now include massage and reflexology as part of the recovery process in patients while the Department of Health have given some GPs the go-ahead to refer their patients to osteopaths. Paying for these treatments privately is expensive, so do check with your GP to see if you might be eligible for treatment on the NHS. Osteopathy in particular can be used to help everyone from babies with colic to the elderly suffering from arthritis. Personally, when I've visited my osteopath I feel wonderfully revived.

STRESS

The flip side of not pampering ourselves enough and not taking the time out to relax and unwind is the danger of stress. Stress is one of the curses of living in the Nineties. As we work longer hours and worry about our finances, and the threat of redundancy, so stress takes its toll. Doctors report that more and more people are taking time off work due to stress-related illnesses than ever before and it's

TOP TIPS

- Organize yourself so that you don't need to rush – make a list if necessary. I always make a point of getting everywhere on time and therefore I'm not stressed when I arrive.
- If people are asking too much of you then put your foot down. Don't let your work colleagues or your family put undue pressure on you.
- At work, accept changes with an open mind and always prioritize.
- Don't try to do too much. No one expects you to be a superwoman. If you are exhausted and the hall carpet needs hoovering then leave it. It will still be there tomorrow.
- Pamper yourself. Reserve a little time every day, even if it's only for 20 minutes, to read a chapter of your favourite book, listen to a play on the radio or complete a crossword.
- Consider burning off stress by doing some physical activity. Take the dog for a walk or take a trip down the local shop for a pint of milk and allow the cobwebs to blow away.
- Don't bottle problems up – talk to someone.

something that affects everyone from the old age pensioner who frets about eking out a living on her state pension to the young mum who worries about her large mortgage. Some people thrive on stress and I know that I will often perform better if I am a little hyped up, but that is different from letting the day-to-day pressures of life grind you down. There is nothing wrong with admitting that you are stressed out and if you feel that life is becoming too pressured I would strongly recommend that you consult a doctor or get counselling. As the body is not designed to cope with the physical effects of stress on a regular basis – such as tensing of the muscles and increased heartbeat – the result of untreated stress can mean extra pressure on the vital organs and possibly disease. Therefore a day-to-day mental problem may become a physical one too, resulting in anything from high blood pressure to asthma, impotence and ulcers.

There are many levels of stress, from feeling just mildly anxious to a full-scale breakdown, but recognizing the causes early on may save you from reaching a critical stage later on.

Sleeping

Not being able to sleep can become a major source of stress to many people. It is believed that the body uses the time when we are asleep to restore and revive itself. By getting a good seven hours' sleep a night we allow our muscles to recover and as our metabolism slows down, our immune system gets the chance to repair damage and fight infections. It is said that we need less and less sleep as we get older and it's estimated that the elderly need the least of all – as little as five hours is adequate. I don't currently find that to be the case, possibly because I lead such an active life. A few years ago I suffered from sleepless nights and was taking all sorts of prescribed sleeping pills which I hated. These days I'm luckier and never have any problems getting to sleep at night. I do sometimes find myself waking up early in the morning which can be irritating, but I don't allow sleeplessness to become a big issue. One thing I always do at the studio is have a short nap during my lunch hour as we record in the evening and I need all my energy then. It doesn't have to be for very long – I close my eyes and sometimes realize that I've only been asleep for a couple of minutes, but I feel instantly revived. I remember someone saying to me once that half an hour in the afternoon is the most beneficial sleep of all. An hour is too long, but half an hour is just enough for the body to repair itself in preparation for the hours to come before bedtime. It is particularly helpful if you're going to be working hard in the afternoon or having a late night.

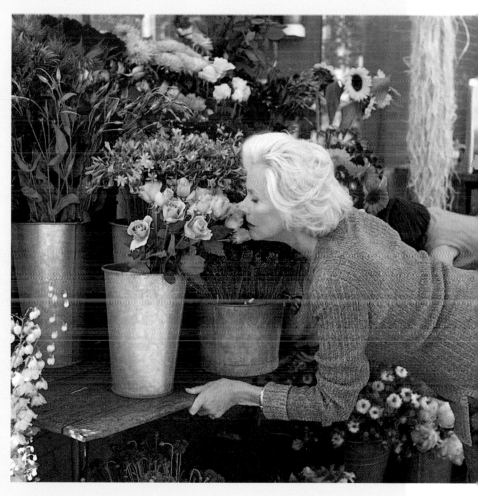

If insomnia is a problem for you, think about cutting down on tea, coffee and alcohol. Also avoid heavy meals late at night, don't succumb to long naps during the day and if you can't sleep then get up and have a bath or a cup of camomile tea. Try to get back to basics and re-establish a night-time routine.

Mmm – heavenly! I find that flowers provide an instant uplift.

Depression

If you find that your stress has not been helped by any of the self-help measures you have tried you may be suffering from depression, in which case you really should seek some professional help. Everyone feels a bit low from time to time but true depression may affect your concentration, appetite and sleeping patterns and leave you suffering feelings of utter despair. Depression is not a sign of weakness and it's not always the result of a major event like a death or loss of job. Even if you don't need or want medication, a doctor or counsellor will be able to help you with ways to relax and feel positive about life again.

Smoking

Women who smoke often use the excuse that it helps them to cope with stress and keeps their weight down. I used to smoke around 20 cigarettes a day but sometimes, if I was filming, it might creep up to 30 or more. I smoked right up until about 15 years ago. When I decided to give up I went to a hypnotist a couple of times who did seem to be rather good, but I didn't persist. When I eventually gave up I did it completely by myself – I went cold turkey, if you like. I was due to go to Canada to work and I said 'When I come back I will not be smoking' and I wasn't.

Let nobody tell you that you have to put on a lot of weight as a result of quitting. You will if you stuff yourself in order to compensate for the absence of nicotine, but if you have any sense you'll be watching what you eat and not consuming too many fatty things. I don't know what I used as a substitute – but I did know of the dangers of compensating in other areas. People constantly said to me that I was marvellous for doing it, but the time was obviously right. Smoking is the single most damaging thing you can do to your health. It's particularly bad for women, who may suffer from fertility problems, cancer of the cervix or heart attacks, particularly if they take the contraceptive pill as well. You don't need me to tell you how dangerous and harmful smoking is but do consider giving up for the sake of your health and your children. The children of smokers tend to have more chest infections and ear problems than those of non-smokers, and smoking has also been linked to cot death.

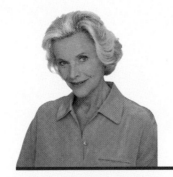

'Going "cold turkey" is the only way to give up smoking – it was how I managed to do it.'

SELF-HELP

I'm very hot on the principle of self help – to me it's a form of pampering. If I want to make sure that I work well as a whole then I ensure that each individual part of me is well maintained and cared for. We are like machines – you wouldn't expect your car to work properly if you didn't service it and the body is no different. On a daily basis I always try to eat a well-balanced diet and aim to get the majority of my vitamins and minerals from food. To make up any shortfall in my supply I also see a naturopath called Julia Barnes who treats me with a balance of herbs and vitamins. I've just recently started taking a supplement called Maxi Multi which, according to Julia, includes all the vitamins and minerals that I require. In order to stave off memory loss and mental disintegration, a good memory being more vital to an actor than to almost anybody else, she advises something called Ginkgo plus; which is a Chinese preparation designed to feed the memory tree - how poetic. Julia swears that it slowed down the advance of memory loss in her mother. 'I treat the whole person by taking a detailed medical history and then suggesting particular herbs to balance the body,' Julia explains. When I feel that I need an extra lift I take ginseng, which gives me an instant energy boost.

I try to keep an open mind as far as complementary and holistic medicine are concerned. I'm interested in alternative treatments and remedies and take the time to read up on the latest developments. I'm happy to combine conventional medical practices with natural healing. Since the menopause I've been on hormone replacement therapy (HRT). It's a low dose, so I don't experience a monthly bleed, and I'm happy enough

TOP TIPS:
FOR A GOOD NIGHT'S SLEEP

- Have a relaxing bath, clean your teeth, set the alarm clock and basically set the scene for bedtime.
- Go to bed at a regular time each night (well before midnight) and force yourself to get up at the same time each morning. Don't be tempted to lie in bed for half the morning.
- Make sure your room is warm, comfortable, dark and quiet and that your mattress is comfortable.
- Buy ear plugs if you are distracted by outside noise, or an eye mask if a street light annoys you.
- Put a drop of lavender oil on your pillow to aid sleep.
- Take some deep breaths and try to clear your mind of worries and responsibilities. Try focusing on a future plan or something that pleases you and just let your mind drift into sleep.
- The worst thing about not sleeping is lying there getting into a fret because you're not sleeping. Don't worry – just try to empty your mind totally. When it happens to me I clear the mind and just imagine that I am floating up to the clouds and everything is very peaceful.
- Some people swear by relaxation exercises, so you could also try putting awareness into each part of your body, starting at the toes. By the time you get to your head you'll have nodded off.

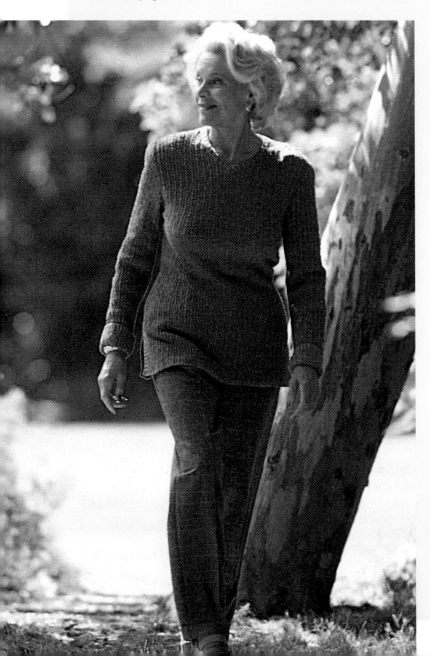

I've been blessed with good health but still give nature a helping hand.

with it. Some women report that HRT gives them a tremendous energy boost, but I haven't particularly noticed this myself. When I cut it out for six months as a test I didn't notice any difference in my energy levels, but we all react differently. If you are suffering because of the menopause, see my Top Tips on the opposite page for a few things you can do to help yourself. It's thought that HRT can also help prevent osteoporosis, lower the risk of heart disease and even ward off the approach of memory lose. Osteoporosis (also known as brittle bones) can affect one in four women after the onset of the menopause, when the reduction in oestrogen levels leads to the loss of bone mass. You may be prone to it if it's in the family genes, if you are underweight or if you drink and smoke a lot. Help to build healthy bones by eating a balanced diet rich in Vitamin D and calcium. Oily fish (like mackerel and herrings) and fortified breakfast cereals contain Vitamin D, while milk (even skimmed), bread, beans and green vegetables are full of calcium. HRT doesn't suit all women, but your doctor will be able to advise you accordingly if the menopause is proving problematic.

Helping myself also means regular check-ups and self-examination. Breast cancer kills more women than any other form of cancer in England. I check my breasts every month not only for lumps but for any change in the shape or the outline of the breast, any puckering or dimpling of the skin or change in the nipple position. Because I am aware of the dangers I would have no hesitation at all in visiting my doctor the moment I thought something was wrong. I can't understand women who find something abnormal and are too frightened to do anything about it – surely it's better to get any problems sorted out immediately before the condition gets dangerously worse? I was certainly glad that I had had regular cervical smears when some abnormal cells were found during a routine smear test. The minute I knew that something was wrong I had the appropriate treatment immediately – I can't bear suspense and would have gone wild not knowing what the problem was. I've had laser treatment and believe that everything is now fine. Going along for a cervical smear, usually every three to five years, is vital. The test is quick and painless and can usually be done by the practice nurse if you are embarrassed about a male GP performing it. If abnormal cells are found then they can be treated almost immediately and the success rate is very high. Major surgery is rarely needed and early treatment will not affect either your sex drive or your fertility. Cervical cancer can affect both young and older women, and indeed the incidence is increasing among the younger generation.

TREAT YOURSELF

I know that having a full life can often mean that we neglect ourselves. Many of us are so busy running around after other people and making sure that they are happy that we tend to forget our own needs. But I always make a point of having quiet times too. If you enjoy watching a particular television programme or going for a walk on your own, then do it. If everybody else in the house complains, well, they'll just have to accept that you need some 'me' time too. Thirty minutes out of every day dedicated to what you want to do isn't too much to ask and you'll feel revived and happy as a result. That is what a little pampering is all about.

TOP TIPS

- Cut down on alcohol, spicy food, tea and coffee if they make your hot flushes worse.
- Keep your bedroom cool and have a cold drink at the side of the bed in case of night sweats.
- Keep active.
- Find out if there is a Well Woman clinic in your area and go and chat to a female doctor. No matter how sympathetic a man may be, women are much more experienced in this area.

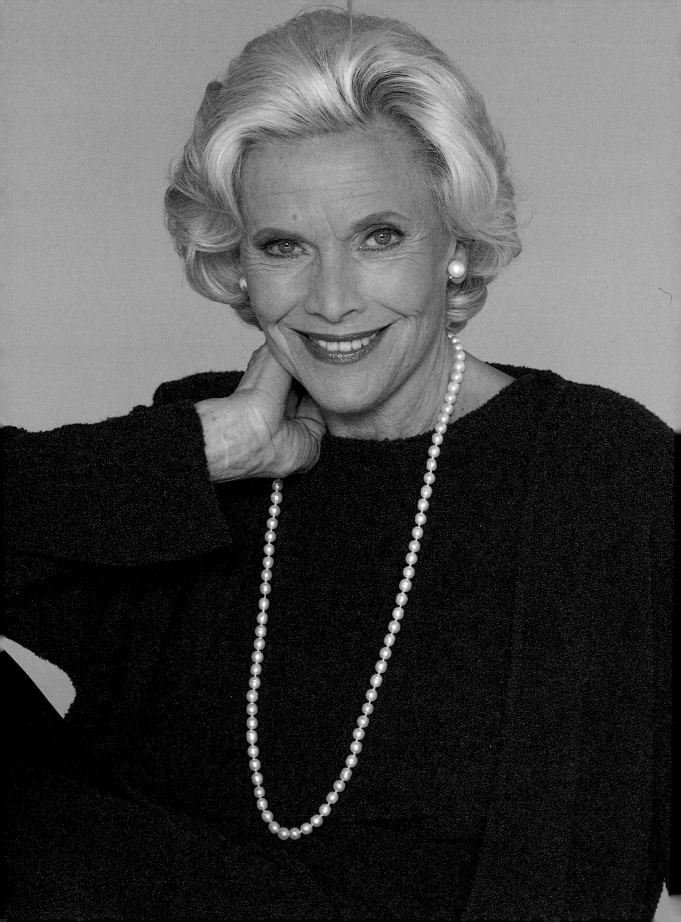

STYLE: TIMELESS ELEGANCE

There is a line from a famous song that goes 'You've either got or you haven't got style'. Well, believe me, when I started out I didn't have a clue about stylish dressing. I was hopeless about putting clothes together and certainly didn't have a particular look. What has happened in the meantime is that I've been knocked into shape by the costume designers who've been responsible for making me look good on stage and screen. They have said yes or no to outfits on my behalf or put me into things without even asking me if I liked them. Consequently, I now have a pretty good idea about what I should wear for any occasion. Over the years I've got to know my figure faults and learnt what suits me and what doesn't. I think I'm lucky in that I've been very well trained.

I look best in trousers and long dresses because I'm an hourglass shape and when you have a fair-sized bust anything that gives you length is more flattering – my bust used to be huge but now, thank the Lord, I have lost some of it, which is a blessing. In addition I've got slim legs, big-boned hips, no bottom and generally no tummy. I often find it difficult to buy clothes to fit me because, I suspect like most women, I'm not a standard size. I have particular trouble buying anything cut by European designers – if the bottom of a suit fits I have extreme difficulty in doing the jacket up.

I like to wear trousers which are pleated at the waist because it means that my hips are not accentuated. Just as a broad person should avoid horizontal stripes and a short person should steer clear of flouncy, flared clothes, so for me, the longer my body looks from shoulder to waist the better. That way my bosom isn't shunted into my waist.

CONTENTS

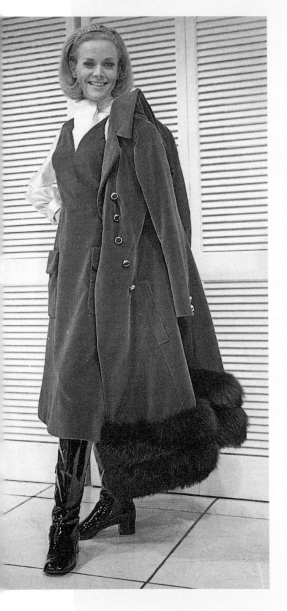

I wore this delicious Dior ensemble in *Who Killed Santa Claus?*

FASHION

I don't give a hoot for fashion. What comes in one season and disappears the next doesn't affect how I look in the slightest. I aim to dress classically, and I think I always have done. I was sorting out some photographs recently and came across a picture of myself in 1968. It was at an evening event and I was wearing a pair of tailored black crepe trousers and a matching single-breasted jacket – exactly the kind of thing I would consider wearing today. The look hasn't dated in the slightest. I like clothes in which I can move freely and feel comfortable. I remember one time when I borrowed a dress from Dior; I discovered on going to the ladies room that I had to take the whole thing off before I could use the lavatory. The attendant to helped me to wriggle out - we became friends!

All the cropped T-shirts and Doc Martens in the world are never going to appeal to me and I couldn't care less what the supermodels are getting up to. I think that fashions and trends are aimed more at women in their twenties and as the years go by we should each develop a style of our own and dress according to our shape and colouring, rather than simply following what the catwalks are dictating – if we've got any sense.

When we are young we don't mind saving up for an outrageous outfit from a trendy high street store which we'll wear all summer and then discard when it falls to pieces, but I've long passed that stage. I favour investment dressing. Being a slave to fashion or, worse, becoming a fashion victim is really quite sad – just look at Jennifer Saunders' character in *Absolutely Fabulous* for confirmation of that.

One sees so many women dressed ultra fashionably who look just dreadful. They have obviously paid a fortune for their outfit because it is 'in' and has the right label, but it simply doesn't suit them. I'm not suggesting for a minute that we have to look boring – it's simply a matter of re-evaluating from time to time what we can get away with. I still see a lot of women who seem to have got stuck in an Eighties time warp and insist upon wearing power suits with skirts up to who-knows-where. They've often got dreadful legs and shouldn't have done it – even in the Eighties.

KEEP IT CLEAN

When I am choosing clothes I always go for understatement. I like very clean lines and simple styles, otherwise the look becomes fussy. With a full bust the last thing I want is anything too busy. For daytime I like to wear silk shirts – I've got a whole range of colours from designer stores and high street shops like Marks & Spencer. I maintain that silk shirts are a classic investment; they last for years, never go out of fashion and always look stylish. I'll team up my shirts with a pair of beautifully cut trousers in black, taupe or sand. It's a very easy look to put together and means that I never find myself scrabbling in the wardrobe for something to wear. By knowing what suits me and sticking to it, I can simply select any of my coloured shirts which I have chosen to complement my trousers and I'm dressed and ready to go in a matter of minutes.

I don't think that style is about having hundreds of designer outfits to hand or a bottomless pit of money available to spend on clothes. True style is simply knowing what is right for you and when to wear it, and this gives you confidence. In the evening, my rule for simple styles still applies. You'll never see pictures of me floating around in a frothy ballgown or done up in anything covered in swathes of net and lace.

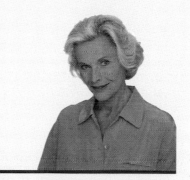

'I always buy the best that I can afford as I consider my clothes to be an investment.'

I love to look glamorous and I love to look sexy, and these aims are achieved by choosing evening dresses that will flatter my figure and hide my imperfections – I have one dress designed by Jasper Conran which is the perfect example of this. One of my favourite designers from *The Upper Hand* is Jimmie Dark. At one time not long ago, Jimmie and I were looking at clothes for a new series when he spotted a wonderful dress in Harvey Nichols in London. We wanted something long-sleeved, black and very sexy and this was just perfect. Jimmie asked the assistant to put it to one side and I went with him the next day to try it on. Because it contains Lycra the dress is very fitted, and it is studded all over with tiny chipped beads, giving it an understated sparkle. I loved it on sight but trying it on was

TOP TIPS

When I'm shopping either for myself or for television I like to visit the main department stores as well a selection of specialist shops. I'll always try on the labels I have bought in the past because I know that these will fit and flatter me. I find it difficult to buy trousers because I have a long 'rise' (this is the length between the crotch and waist), so tried and tested styles are the first I'll go for. I look for good cut, good quality and affordability. I don't spend a fortune on my clothes and designer labels are not my highest priority. If I like a particular outfit, know that I'll wear it and consider it to be a reasonable price, then I may consider buying it. What I do like to have is a selection of outfits that will see me through a number of different occasions. In some ways it's often easier to dress for a glamorous evening event; if you have a classic black dress then you can dress it up with some glitzy jewellery and you are off.

another matter. I managed to get it over my head but it was a pretty scratchy process. When it was on we both realized it was a knock-out. I paid a lot of money for it but have worn it constantly since – it's what I call a 'go out and perform dress'. When I'm 'on duty' it is perfection as the effect it has on my confidence is phenomenal.

COLOURS

Because my hair is fair and my skin tone is light I choose shades which complement my natural colouring. I generally avoid garish colours and loud patterns because I don't want my clothes to take over. When I buy a blouse or evening dress I'll usually select one that will work as an extension of me, but on the occasions when I do wear a rather dashing blouse I'll make sure that it is the only garish item I'm wearing. Taupes, soft yellows and greys and all very earthy tones work well for me, or in sharp contrast, if I am going out for the evening, I'll go for something strong like midnight blue or black, both of which are flattering. I've found that in the day black can be very draining so I tend to avoid it, but at night when I'm all dressed up with a little sparkly jewellery I know that I can get away with it.

The way that I've organized my wardrobe and purchased new items over recent years gives me the choice of many outfits, because each item goes with at least two or three others. I've tried to work on the principle of mix and match.

Knowing which colours suit me is mainly a result of trial and error and taking advice from designers. If you are uncertain about what to choose there are now a number of companies in business, including Colour Me Beautiful, who for the price of a consultation will be able to advise you on what you should wear. Although this may seem an expensive luxury, it may help you save money by avoiding the wrong choices in future. Alternatively, go through your wardrobe and select

Right: Grey jersey wool cardigan and T-shirt with grey wool trousers. The soft textures of clothes like these are heaven to wear. The twinset is wonderfully comfortable yet stylish too. I would wear this if I was working on a script or lyrics at home. By adding something as exotic as this Turkish jewellery, this outfit can be dressed up or down.

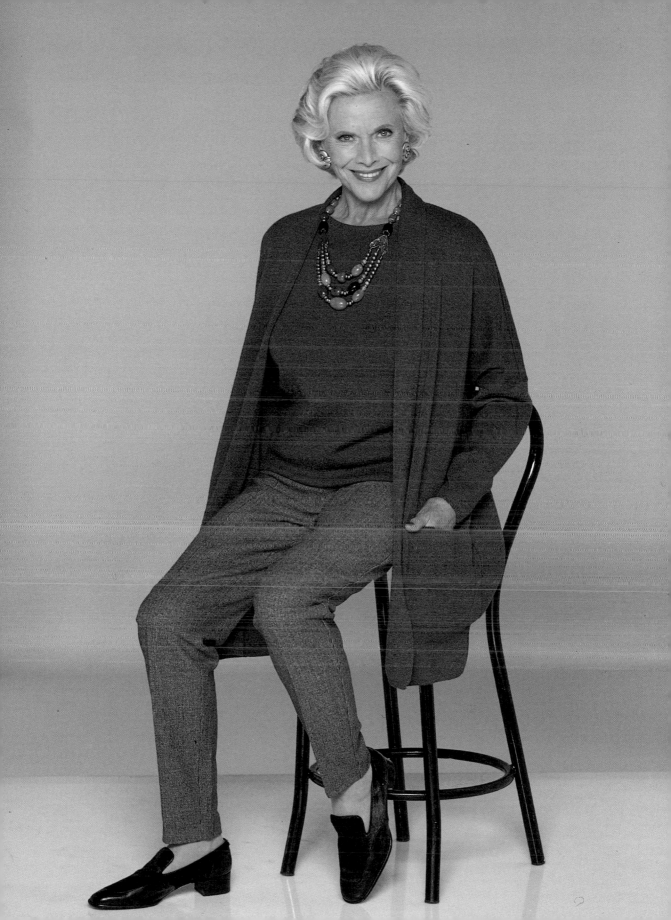

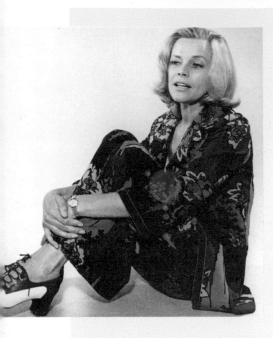

One of my favourite outfits of all time. I've still got this Annacat suit – it's simply cut and a joy to wear.

Right: Cossack coat. Something like this fabulous coat is the ultimate in investment dressing. It will cost a lot of money but will last for at least 10 years and will never go out of fashion. Before investing you would have to make sure that you are going to get good wear out of it and if you drive everywhere you probably won't. Nevertheless, wearing something like this makes me feel like Anna Karenina herself!

six or seven items all in different colours. Sit in front of your mirror in good natural light and hold each of the colours in turn under your chin. That way you'll see which of them compliments your skin, hair and eyes best. You'll notice that some shades will make your skin tone look fresh and bright, while others will render it dull. Some colours will enhance your eyes, while others will do little for you. Only by taking the time and trouble to sit down and work out what suits you will you be able to make the right choices next time you shop. Most shops and department stores are lit with fluorescent strip lights that distort colours, and something that suits you under such lighting may look hideous worn in the cold light of day. Don't be shy about taking your chosen garment over to the window to check its true shade – don't be intimidated if it's implied you are being fussy, but do tell the assistant what you are doing first! Always have a clear idea about your good points and limitations before you leave home as that way you may be able to cut down on the number of bad buys you make.

TAKE STOCK

Most of us have bulging wardrobes, yet often the cry is 'I haven't got a thing to wear'. In most cases you probably have got plenty of things to wear, it's just a matter of getting organized. In my apartment I have a huge wardrobe and I make a real effort to de-junk and reorganize regularly. Here's how you can do it too.

- *Invite an honest friend around for the evening and set to work. Empty the entire content of your wardrobe onto the bedroom floor and sort it out.*
- *Then create three separate piles of clothes: one for the must-keeps, one for the maybes and one for the charity shop.*
- *Try to be realistic — if you haven't worn those size 10 stretch jeans at all in the last five years then you're never likely to again, are you?*
- *Try on all of the must-keeps first and edit them down further if need be. You may have to accept that some old favourites have simply worn out, and unless you plan to have them copied it's better to throw them away.*

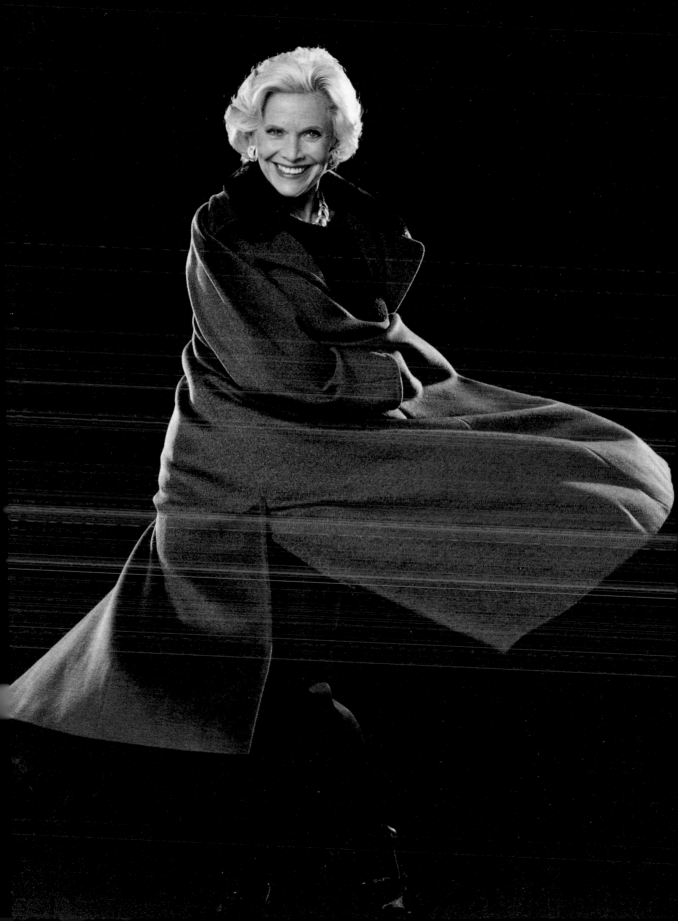

- *Now try on all the 'maybes' and unless you like what you see and have worn each item at least twice in the past two years, edit this pile down too.*
- *Once you have decided what you are keeping and losing, rearrange your remaining wardrobe. Organize your clothes in types, so that all blouses are together, all jackets are together and so on — that way you'll know at a glance what is available to wear.*
- *Don't put anything back that needs washing, dry cleaning or mending (the same applies to shoes and underwear).*
- *Hang your clothes on proper hangers, not those cheap wire ones that give you points in your shoulders. If you can't afford padded or wooden ones, wrap tissue paper around wire ones.*
- *Once you have organized your wardrobe you will be able to see where there are gaps in your clothes and you'll know what you need to budget for.*

TIME FOR CHANGE

I believe that once we get away from the concept of dressing fashionably and start dressing stylishly then we begin to look our very best and relax into a style of our own. Nearly all the smart women I know came into their own when they hit a certain age and started dressing in exactly what suited them. It's hard for all of us to accept that we aren't the young girl that we once were but harking back to our youth and to how we used to look and dress is pointless. As we get older we change and gain a certain sophistication – just look at women like Princess Diana. The shape of our bodies changes, especially after childbirth, our complexions tone down and our hair often subtly changes colour too. In the last 15 years mine has gone from blonde to brown, which is maddening because silver would mix with blonde more easily. Once we recognize such changes taking place then it's time to think again about where we shop, what we buy and how much we spend. Skirt lengths are a typical example of this. There are not many women who can get away with micro skirts and still look elegant. I've always maintained that there is a good part to the leg – usually just on the knee – and the shape frequently deteriorates from there up.

Your skirt length should be long enough to hide any bulging thighs or dimpled knees and short enough to show off

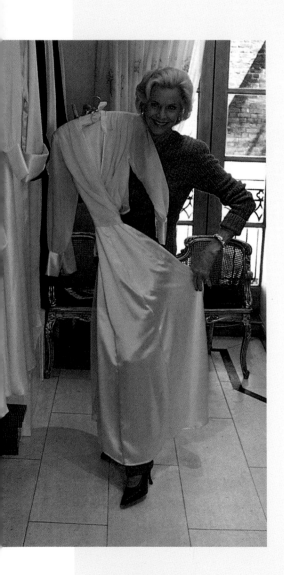

Who could resist this pretty silk peignoir from Janet Reger?

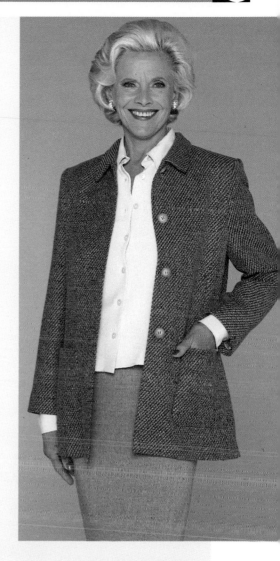

shapely calves and slim ankles. Skirts that are too short on bad legs or contain too little fabric look cheap, and those that stretch tightly around your backside like a rubber band simply look tarty. Looking stylish means recognizing your limits. I've always thought the same applies with swimsuits. Wearing a swimsuit with a high leg can be flattering up to a point, but if it is cut too high you haven't got long legs any more – you've simply got big hips. You've lived with your body for long enough, you know what your limitations are, so be honest with yourself.

CLEVER INVESTMENTS

Investment dressing isn't cheap, but if you are shrewd your purchases should last a lifetime. As a young woman you may have spent £40 on a trendy jacket from a flashy boutique; now you may have to accept the fact that you need to pay nearer £100 for a classic version from a more grown-up store, but ideally you'll be purchasing something made of better fabric with more detailed finishing. I've still got clothes in my wardrobe which I've had for years and still wear. Something like a simple cashmere sweater or a pair of pure wool tapered trousers may cost a lot initially but they will be timelessly elegant. There are certain clothes that no wardrobe should be without and you'll wear them time after time:

- *Little black dress – spend as much as you can afford on a scoop-necked, knee-length black dress. It will take you anywhere. You will be able to dress it up with glitzy jewellery and wear it on countless occasions. If you can find a full-length version, buy that too – you won't regret it.*

- *A basic suit – at least one. Preferably in black, brown or charcoal grey, it will prove extremely versatile and durable. If the jacket comes with a choice of skirt and trousers then all the better – you'll be able to mix and match all three pieces with other things in your wardrobe. If you buy a basic suit from a chain store, stamp your own personality on it by buying designer-style buttons from a department store and replacing the originals.*

- *Good trousers – beautifully cut, in navy or taupe, for wearing with shirts or sweaters. Wonderful material is important, and make sure they are lined.*

Above: Cream crepe shirt, grey suiting skirt and soft, single-breasted wool jacket. This is something that Jimmie always calls the 'hands in pockets look' and it's the kind of outfit I would wear to a casual lunch with a friend out of town. I put this look together by first selecting the blouse, which flatters my skin tone, and then layering other colours on top. With this look I would wear a pair of soft suede shoes with a heel and choose a bag that co-ordinates rather than matches exactly. Simple earrings complete the effect.

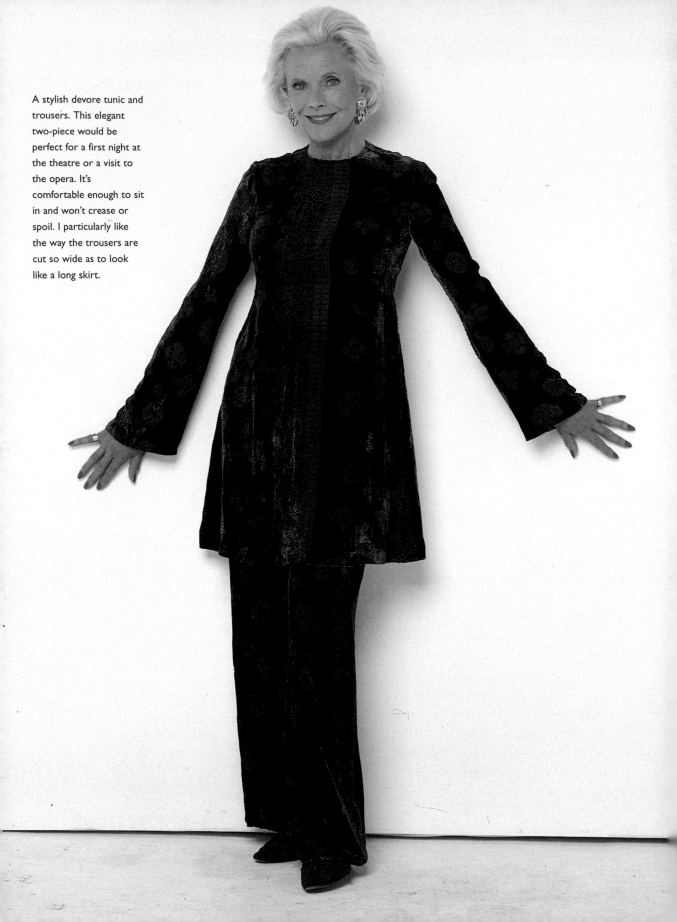

A stylish devore tunic and trousers. This elegant two-piece would be perfect for a first night at the theatre or a visit to the opera. It's comfortable enough to sit in and won't crease or spoil. I particularly like the way the trousers are cut so wide as to look like a long skirt.

- *Something fun like a Spanish skirt — I love skirts that whoosh at the bottom because I like movement and clothes that swing. It's the nearest I get to frills and trimmings.*

- *Shirts — I'm a great fan of silk. Also invest in one classic white cotton shirt which will look equally good with a smart suit or light 'chino' style trousers or 501 jeans at weekends.*

- *Cotton 'bodies' — invest in a selection of colourful shades for wearing under separates. They also double up well under a sarong on holiday.*

- *Shoes — although we all own a jumble of shoes, basically you only need three pairs, low, medium and high, and if they are all black you can't go wrong. I also like to have a lightweight pair of stone or cream sandals or shoes to wear with cottons on sunny days.*

- *A classic raincoat in navy or beige will never date. Supplement this with a black wool shawl for evenings.*

SMART MONEY

I'm not a bitty dresser; I invest in the essentials but I ultimately believe that less is more. Vital are a couple of narrow, smart leather belts, one in black and one in brown, that go with everything. Two handbags are quite sufficient; one large black leather one for daytime — I try to de-junk mine regularly — and a small black patent one with a long fabric cord strap for evenings (this can either be worn over the shoulder or the cord can be tucked inside and the bag used as a clutch). Sunglasses are a must too, both in summer and in winter on sunny days. Not only will they protect your eyes from dust and pollution but they'll also stop you from squinting against the light and exacerbating crow's feet round your eyes.

I don't spend a fortune on lingerie. I have been to Janet Reger and Harvey Nichols for

TOP TIPS WHEN SHOPPING

- Have a plan. Twice a year, in September and March, check through last year's clothes and see what will still be wearable for the six months ahead. Then decide what you need to buy in addition to create a working wardrobe. That way you'll avoid expensive mistakes.

- Set a budget but don't tie yourself completely to it. If you are looking for a perfect black jacket and find it at a price, buy it rather than opting for a cheaper, inferior version. I'll guarantee that you'll wear it for years.

- Before you go out, stand naked in front of the mirror and take a long critical look at what you see and how your shape may have changed. Think about the types of clothes you've felt happy wearing recently and bear this in mind when choosing something new.

- Never impulse-buy anything major if you are in a rush. If you see something you like, try it on and ask the assistant if you can put it aside until the next day. Go home and check through your wardrobe. If it won't work with at least three other garments in there, forget it. I recently went out shopping for a pair of practical shoes to wear to rehearsals. My car was on a parking meter and time was ticking away, and in my haste I bought a pair of expensive high-heeled evening shoes made of satin and net from a Bond Street store. I got them home and realized they are far too narrow for me (I've got rather wide feet) and they absolutely kill me — so buying in haste is madness.

- Try to be strong. If you're not sure about something, don't allow an eager shop assistant to persuade you. I find the more they push the more I back off.

- If you find something you really like, buy two. From a pair of perfectly fitting shoes to a comfortable bra, the chances are you may not be able to find them again.

- Reassess your needs. You may once have been a high-flying executive who needed sharp suits and court shoes, but if you are now a busy mum running a company from home you'll need softer styles in more comfortable fabrics. You'll want clothes that can be thrown in the washing machine rather than dragged off to the dry cleaners every time your youngster dribbles on you.

- Be prepared to change according to your lifestyle and needs at each stage of your life.

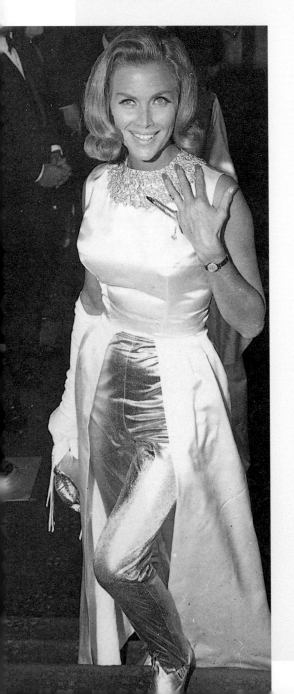

At the première of
Goldfinger – complete
with gold finger!

particular items like camisoles but I do go to Marks & Spencer too. I prefer natural fibres like cotton and silk. One item I don't stint on, ever, is my bra. I think it's vital to have a properly fitted bra at all times and I've paid up to £100 for mine before now. A marvellous mail order firm called Bravissimo specialize in bras for the generously endowed. I would have been most grateful to them earlier in my career! I remember being taken to a corset maker for a bra fitting when I was very young. In those days you couldn't buy ready-to-wear bras – they had to be made to measure, and I paid over £40 even then!

Another area where I pay particular attention is in the purchasing of hosiery. I ruthlessly throw away any stockings or tights that are past their best and always keep a fresh pair in my handbag in case of accidents. The new lacy and opaque styles from companies like Fogal and Wolford do tend to be expensive but they last for ages and are terribly slimming on the leg – especially those which contain Lycra. I also particularly like wearing 'hold-ups' as I find them very cool, and healthy, too.

DRESSING TO IMPRESS

One of the perks of working on stage and in TV is that I get to wear some wonderful clothes. Like many actresses on TV I am able to buy some of the clothes my character has worn, and luckily for me Laura West from *The Upper Hand* has good taste. In the earliest part of my career, when I was under contract to Rank, I played lots of fresh-faced virgin types with modest attire to match. Later, when I began to play more meaty roles, I did nothing but display my bust. However, one of the most fondly remembered creations I ever wore was to the première of *Goldfinger* in 1964. My dressmaker, Jay Terry, created a white duchess satin top embroidered with very fine gold frogging and gold lamé trousers. It was a beautiful outfit, but I realized at the eleventh hour that the trousers alone would not be formal enough for such a prestigious event. I rang Jay and told him I needed him to add a half skirt to match the top. Although he cursed me he came up with the goods, and the effect was wonderful. I also wore a gold finger on my left hand. It was a nightmare. The finger had been designed by the

American jeweller Charles de Temple, had a 6.5 carat diamond hanging from it and was worth $10,000 then. For insurance purposes it was decided that I had to have two burly security men with me at all times when I was wearing it – even when I went to the ladies room. After the usual rounds of promotional work for the film you can imagine that I got mightily fed up with being followed at every turn. Did I get to keep the finger? You must be joking! In fact, I have absolutely no idea what happened to it. I seem to be rather unlucky as far as film jewellery goes. I died a particularly gruesome death in the 1968 film *Shalako* when I was choked to death with diamonds. In that film I had to have my outer garments torn off me by a group of Apache Indians. Because the clothes were so well made and no one had clipped the French seams they simply weren't tearing off me. By the time I was finally reduced to my camisole actual pieces of my flesh had been removed. Diamonds are not this girl's best friend!

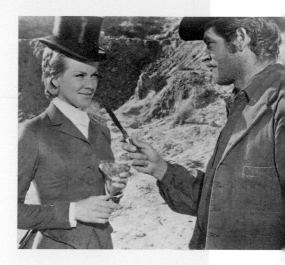

With Stephen Boyd in *Shalako*, a film I did not escape from unscathed.

I think the most glamorous clothes I wore on stage were those by Christian Dior for the play *Who Killed Santa Claus?* at the Piccadilly Theatre. One ensemble comprised a purple velvet midi-coat banded with wide black fox. Underneath I wore a matching purple pinafore dress with a creamy white satin blouse and Dior patent leather boots – a far cry from the leather outfit of *The Avengers*

THAT SUIT

The first leather suit that I wore in *The Avengers* was green, but in those days of black and white TV that didn't matter. What did matter was that when I wore fabric trousers they had split in a close-up during a fight. It was decided then that this shouldn't be repeated and I was to have a more practical fighting suit in a stronger fabric. Patrick Macnee suggested something in suede but the producer rejected that because suede tends to absorb light. Finally we settled on leather, and my outfit became my uniform for the next two years. It comprised a long-sleeved, round-necked jerkin that buttoned up across the front and a pair of black leather trousers. It was a purely practical effort. Lots of people make the mistake

Right: Brown tweed trouser suit. This classic two-piece looks wonderful with a sage-coloured silk shirt, brown belt and black boots. I might wear this if I were being interviewed in town or attending a working lunch. By dressing up the more conventional tweed with amber earrings and a bright bracelet I make it more sexy. Therefore the whole look is an irresistible contradiction of sex and structure.

Though many people thought it was a catsuit, the outfit I wore in *The Avengers* was a two-piece so that I could move my arms freely.

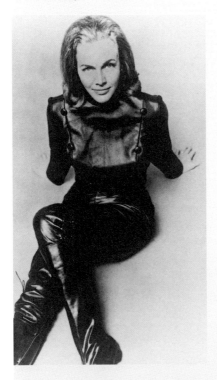

of thinking that it was a catsuit, but a catsuit wouldn't have worked because I needed the freedom to move my arms about when fighting as I had to be able to raise my arms above my head.

I remember that once when I walked into the designer's studio for a fitting there were hundreds of black leather suits hanging up ready for dispatch. 'What are they?' I asked. 'Oh, they are Cathy Gale suits and they are all going into Harvey Nichols' windows next week,' said the designer. 'I doubt that very much,' I replied, and put a block on it. I was furious.that a deal had been struck to commercialize my costume without a single reference to the person who had designed it and made it famous. Besides, Cathy Gale would have appeared far less interesting if half of London was walking round in the same suit.

THOSE KINKY BOOTS

Once the clothes were complete I had to find some suitable footwear. I actually wore lots of different styles in the series including high thigh boots, but flat leather boots were the only ones I could fight in. I still have my fighting boots – they are the only part of my costume I have ever owned. I read some time ago that one of the auction houses was planning to put them up for sale. Well, I don't know whose boots they had, but they certainly weren't mine.

I suppose it's impossible to talk about those kinky boots without mentioning the record that followed. Decca asked us to make a single and I thought it might be fun. Patrick Macnee said that he couldn't sing and had no sense of rhythm whatsoever, but I didn't believe him and persuaded him to have a go.

We had worked all week plus all day on Saturday on the show and went to Decca's recording studio straight after rehearsals, already exhausted. We quickly found that what Patrick had said was true. Finally he mostly talked his lyrics with someone tapping him on the shoulder when he needed to come in. I don't know if he has ever forgiven me for twisting his arm. I only know we got blind drunk afterwards. When the single was released it enjoyed a chequered career. First off it was a flop, then it was a hit, then it was voted the worst record ever made (my children hung their heads in shame) and then it was

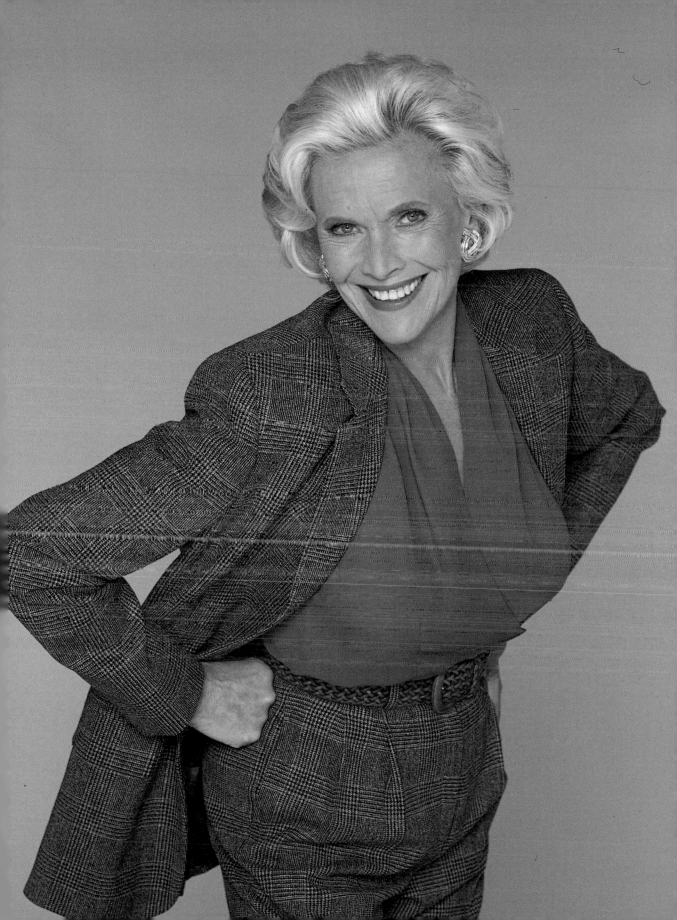

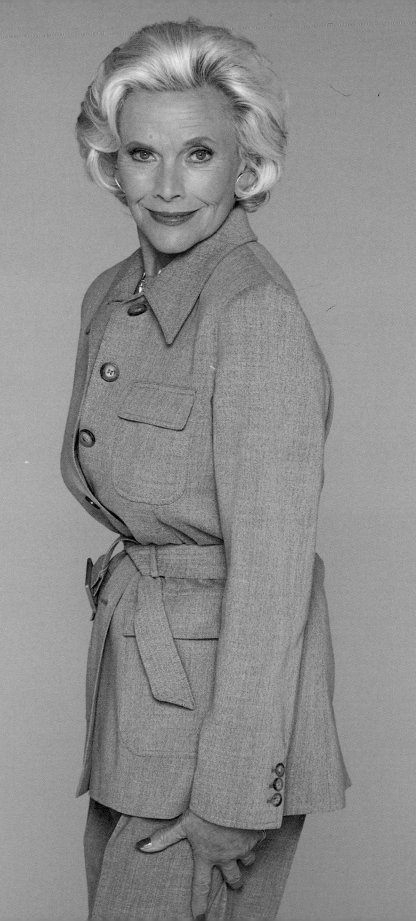

voted a cult hit (they raised them again).

HAIR TODAY

As well as the leather Avengers outfit and those kinky boots, my hairstyle has become something of a trademark. I visit Hugh Green at Hugh and Stephen in London at least every six weeks – I've been going to Hugh for about 15 years and have built up a very good relationship with him. He knows my hair, he knows me and I trust him completely, which is essential. A little while ago my hair looked too blonde on television and was photographing too fair – it looked as if I had a halo, so we discussed it and my colourist Gina toned it down. I've also had the length of it shortened in recent times. I've now gone from the very straight bob I sported in the Sixties to a layered bob, which is softer. It has been cut so that it is fuller at the bottom and layered on top in order to give it lift and a little softness. My hair responds best to being set, and Hugh achieves this by putting my hair in rollers and placing me under a dryer rather than blow-drying it. It is so fine that if I do have it blow-dried it is a mess in minutes and dead straight.

'I would urge every woman to seek out a good hairdresser and build up a trusting relationship,' says Hugh. 'Why spoil what is otherwise a classic wardrobe with scruffy hair? Invest in a few hair magazines, flick through and see which styles you like and which you feel you could cope with yourself considering your lifestyle. Then visit a reputable hairdresser, maybe on a recommendation from a friend, and discuss beforehand what you hope to achieve. A good hairdresser will be happy to discuss the style and offer a few suggestions of his or her own.'

Just like a stylish suit, a good haircut won't come cheap, but you will find that it is worth it. If you have just three classic outfits in your wardrobe, a fresh complexion and a stunning, well-maintained hairstyle you'll be able to go anywhere and meet anyone, looking great and feeling confident.

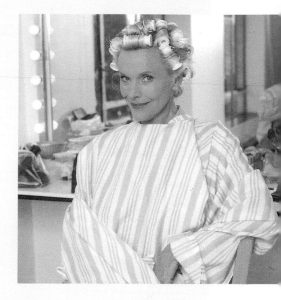

Now here's a shot I bet you never thought you'd see! Rollers aren't glamorous, but for my hair they're best.

Left: Suiting trouser suit. I never like to buckle belts, so I simply tie them like this. The effect is far less formal and a bit of fun. I always think it is important to experiment a little with clothes and find out what works best on you. With some sexy jewellery this instantly becomes a classic suit with a twist.

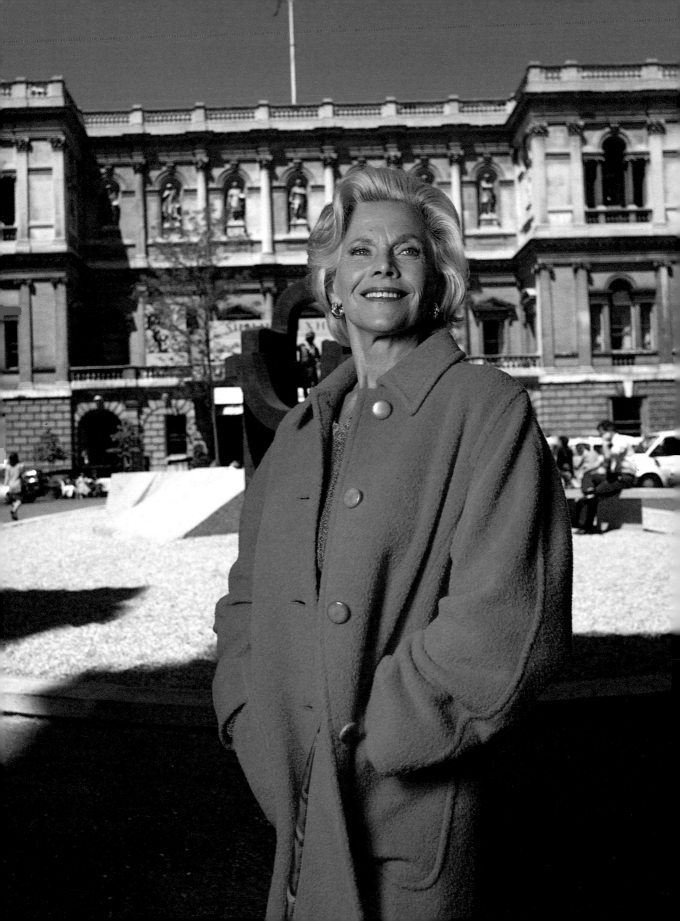

KNOWING YOURSELF AND BEING HAPPY

There is a saying that life is not a rehearsal. Whether it originated in our business I know not, but with that in mind I do try to use my time in as fulfilling a way as possible. I'm a member of the Royal Academy of Arts and a 'Friend' of the Tate, and I enjoy browsing in both galleries and visiting their exhibitions. I used to sit in court and listen to cases being heard, as the law fascinates me. It's quite akin to the acting profession in many ways, with hours of boredom (as in filming), very dramatic moments and people acting their socks off both from the floor and the witness box. It saddens me that I can't go to court as often as I'd like to, but being an onlooker is only fun if you are anonymous and that isn't often the case now.

Of course I go to the theatre and to the movies. Videos at home do not compare with the atmosphere in a darkened cinema with a vast screen. I love walking, and not just in the country or in parks. I know that London is a dirty place as far as pollution is concerned and something must be done to give us an efficient and coordinated public transport system and get us out of our cars, but that aside, there are so many fascinating places in London. The City particularly is a part of town I love to explore, as it's so Dickensian. It takes little imagination to picture the scenes of a century ago.

The river is interesting too, though there are parts up East where I'm nervous of seeing a corpse surface – but then they always give them concrete shoes, don't they? At the end of the run of *The Sound of Music* Petula Clarke and I gave a farewell party for our company on one of the Thames pleasure boats. At night the river is so romantic with the floodlit buildings and the shadows, almost as atmospheric as the Seine, and if you have a band playing, a glass of wine and a lovely partner it can be magical.

CONTENTS

So, I live a full life but not a frantic one. I most certainly try to organize quiet days and nights when I catch up on mail of all kinds, clear up parts of the flat which have become chaotic, and actually do some housework. If I'm worried you'll find me washing the floor.

I wouldn't dream of giving up work until it gives me up – I love it. Of course that's where I'm lucky; my work is interesting, frequently fun and above all varied. Nobody retires us at any given age – they merely dump us when we can't do it any more! But if your job doesn't give you a similar stimulus or you are already retired there are plenty of interests you can involve yourself in, from pottery to amateur dramatics or gardening. You need to have something to look forward to and if you are no good at hobbies there are many voluntary organizations which are crying out for people to help them and where you will feel that you're achieving something for others. If you love to sing then take singing lessons, as I do – you'll so enjoy hearing your improvement. So will your tutor!

I suppose when people ask me how I stay so young what they really mean is I seem so young, since, let's face it, no one does stay young. I imagine it is because I look forward not backward – I enjoy life tremendously and it shows. I eat well and I take exercise and don't hate it. All such things as exercise require some self-discipline. If you over-eat or

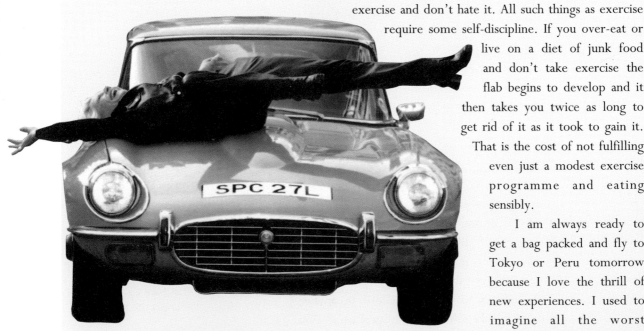

live on a diet of junk food and don't take exercise the flab begins to develop and it then takes you twice as long to get rid of it as it took to gain it. That is the cost of not fulfilling even just a modest exercise programme and eating sensibly.

I am always ready to get a bag packed and fly to Tokyo or Peru tomorrow because I love the thrill of new experiences. I used to imagine all the worst possible scenarios and worry about them ages before they happened. Gradually I've learnt that some of the disasters never materialized and by fretting in anticipation I rendered myself less capable of coping with the problems that did occur. It's taken me a long time to realize that there is no point in worrying about the future if there is nothing practical to be done to control or direct events in advance.

When their families grow up and leave home, many women tend to feel that the most important part of their lives has ended and that memories are all they have left. Well, I feel the complete opposite is true. When my children began to do their own thing I realized that I could reclaim my life and have again the freedom to do all the things that weren't possible while they were still young. With middle age came the opportunity for me to be my own person once more and I gratefully grasped that opportunity with both hands.

LUST FOR LIFE

I have reached a stage in my life when I can honestly say that I am happy. That's a sweeping statement, but it means I like waking up every morning – it doesn't mean there are no problems or that I'm never unhappy, but I do have the confidence that I am unlikely to be overwhelmed by anything that pops up. I am able to take a long view of problems. What

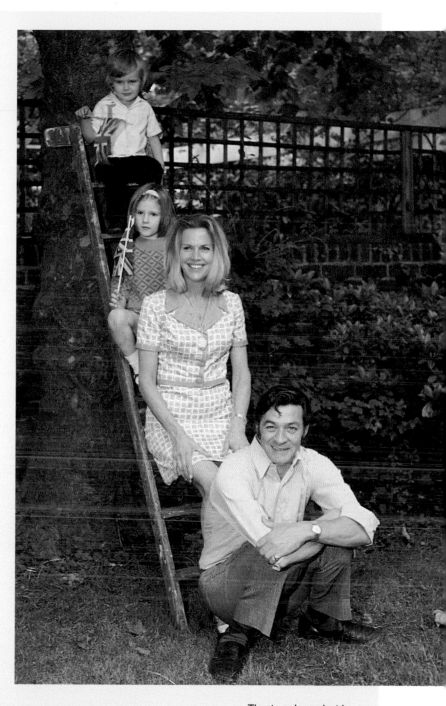

The times I spend with my children have always been the most precious of all. Here we are with Maurice in the Seventies.

MY TOP TIPS FOR A HAPPY LIFE

- Make the most of every new day and make an effort to get up and out.

- Trust your instincts and gut reactions – if you think something is right then go with it.

- Take some time to pamper yourself and pay proper regard to your looks.

- Make time to talk to your partner and enjoy his company.

- If you've got spare time on your hands then take up a new interest. Join a local club or offer your services to a good cause.

- Make an effort to keep in touch with friends.

- Accept that your grown-up children have their own lives and now is the time for you to reclaim yours.

- Have a little compassion for other people. Not everyone is as perfect as you are.

- Take control of the important things in life; pay more attention to your health, diet and general well-being.

- Make sure that you know exactly how much money you have and where it is. Re-evaluate your investments from time to time. Is your money working hard enough for you?

- Have fun, involve yourself with the people who make you laugh. Humour is vitally important at every stage of our lives and laughter is a wonderfully uplifting tonic. I certainly couldn't function without it.

might be a disadvantage or irritation now may with time turn out to be an advantage, and tolerance might be the name of the game. I have accepted that I shall always suffer ghastly nerves in my work, but it's the job I chose and I just have to get on with it, having prepared 100 per cent to ward off disaster.

With this book, my aim has been to put down in black and white how I live my life, my attitude to life and my philosophy, such as it is, and hope that anyone reading it can pick out something from that.

Often I meet very proper middle-aged ladies at the various functions I attend and they'll invariably introduce me to their friends by saying, 'This is the person we would love to be like.' They are referring, of course, to my character Laura West from *The Upper Hand*. I'm sure they don't want to be as sexually promiscuous as she is but they do admire her love of life, the fact that she'll try anything and is interested in everything. I think that's what I have in common with her, a lust for life. The functions I don't enjoy I no longer attend – which might not be good policy for all sorts of reasons, but that's too bad. I have always been fairly forthright and I suspect that now I am even more so. These attitudes can be indulged at this stage of life and there are occasions when they sure lift the pressure.

HOW I LIVE MY LIFE

What makes me happy

On days when I've got some spare time I involve myself with several charities, including Sight Savers, Amnesty Internationl, Action For The Blind and Colon Cancer Campaign. Obviously charities like personalities to become involved with them because it's good for publicity, but anyone can do charity work, whether it's an hour a week spent chatting to longterm patients in the local hospital or helping sort out donated clothes at the charity shop in the high street. Doing my bit gives me enormous satisfaction. I'm also trying to learn to play the piano. I go to lessons whenever I can and have a piano in my apartment for practice, but I admit that my life is so busy sometimes that practice becomes very sporadic. I'm only just beginning but I love friends playing for me as it reminds me of sing-songs around the piano during my childhood.

Music has played a big part in my life. We always had music at home – we would sing and my sister used to play the piano – but it was all popular stuff. I'm not well versed in classical music but I enjoy it, though if you asked me to name my favourite pieces I would fail horribly. On the rare occasions I go to the opera I tend to get very emotional if it's a tragedy. I am often taken by a opera-buff friend who enjoys watching my reactions. If there is something that causes tears to stream down my face he is delighted!

I adore those marvellous American musicals from the Thirties with their super tunes and frequently clever lyrics, which make us leave the theatre on a high and when the orchestra strikes up the overture I find it exciting even when I'm in the show and have played it a hundred times over. I love jazz too, particularly Miles Davis and Thelonious Monk.

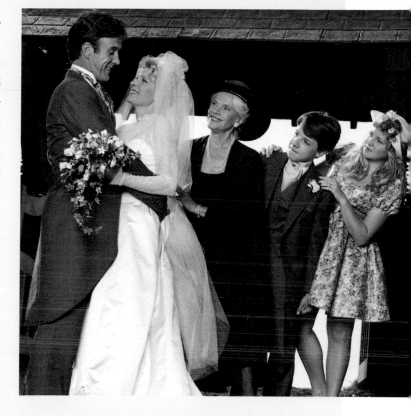

Caroline and Charlie finally tie the knot in *The Upper Hand*. After seven series we've all become good friends.

Friendship

I have a very small circle of very good friends, though of course I know an enormous number of people. I don't suffer from loneliness because if I want to see people I can, but I actually enjoy being alone sometimes for long periods – in fact I think I'd go potty if I were forced to live with someone. But friendships are terribly important. Our best friends are almost always people with similar interests and shared experiences, and it is comforting to talk over family problems and situations with them. There are always friends who'd like a call, a line or a card when they are tense or unhappy, such as when they are about to take a test of some sort or attend a worrying appointment with a doctor. We British are so often reserved and afraid of intruding. My mother used to say 'They will think I'm being pushy', but there are occasions when someone is sitting alone fretting, and wishing that someone *would* push. There's nothing to stop you sharing their joys, either. It took me a long time to discover women friends. When I was a child I was very male-orientated. My father was a strong influence in my life and I suppose I've always cleaved to men. It wasn't until after my marriages that I began to realize that women weren't necessarily rivals and that they could be mates. I'll never forget the time when my daughter Lottie turned down the chance to go on a date with a handsome young man in favour of going out for the evening with a group of girlfriends. 'Why do you want to go out with them when you can go out with him?' I asked. 'Well, Mummy,' she replied, 'boyfriends may come and go but girlfriends last forever.' I was heartened that the realization had struck her so early.

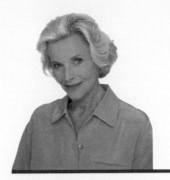

'It took me a long time to realize that other women aren't necessarily rivals and can be valuable friends.'

Often I'll sit with a womanfriend and we'll laugh until we weep about what fools we make of ourselves because we care so much about our children. I'm sorry that I didn't realize sooner in life that females could be such fun.

Family

It's often said that we can choose our friends but we can't choose our families – but just like friendships, family contact has to be worked at too.

Most mothers try to keep out of their children's business but when we have two roles to play, that of carer and protector, it's very difficult to get the balance right. I try desperately not to interfere in my children's lives, except when they ask – that's different. I'm very close to my children Lottie and Barnaby, but family relationships have to be treated with kid gloves. My children say I'm prone to be bossy, which is something I'm very conscious of. I try to control the urge to rearrange other people's lives and it has taken a long time to register that my children, now in their late twenties, have reached the stage when they can say, 'Thanks very much, but my decisions might be better than yours.' Adult offspring obviously know the way they feel better than you, the outsider, do. As children grow older it is only natural that they move away from their parents to develop their own lives. I don't think I've ever had a problem in letting mine go – after all, they've been a couple of rebels from the age of 12. They wanted to be out by themselves long before I thought it was fit but they survived, thank God. Now I realize that they were often quite aware of life's pitfalls and the things that were worrying me were worrying them too.

Sex

Sex isn't only for young people. I believe we can enjoy some of the best sex of our lives when we are older and we know exactly what we want from intimate relationships with no worries about getting pregnant. If sex has become a little stale or routine with your partner, do something about it. I am not in favour of cold-blooded discussions between couples about their needs in bed. Let's be honest, the truth generally comes out when you are hot – either in temper or in bed. A civilized discussion of the subject is clinical. You must know your partner by now, and what turns him on – or used to. Have a plan, but let things appear accidental. Get hold of a romantic video or book that you know he'll find a turn-on. 'Good heavens, I got this book out of the library thinking it was a silly romance, but just read that page!' A drink may be of assistance in creating the right mood, and some sexy clothing – or a lack of it! When he is in a jolly mood, ask him to acquire an erotic film as you have never seen one. Has he? 'Just think, we've got to this stage in our lives and haven't experienced much. I'm curious.'

If you are too shy to go into a

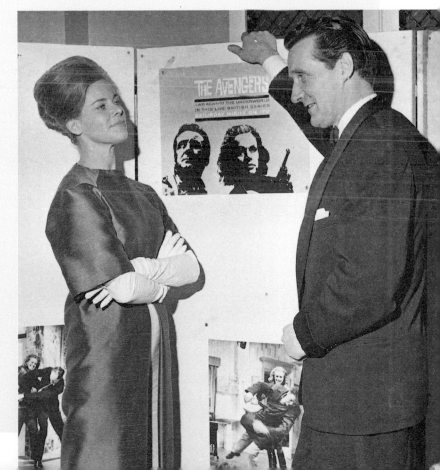

Working with Patrick Macnee (Steed) on *The Avengers* was always enormous fun. His risqué observations still have me in stitches.

local video shop you must have someone among your acquaintances considered a bit of a devil who will get a movie for you if you say you want to gee up your partner. I'm not talking about anything seedy – just something sexy that will get you both aroused.

I remember seeing a blue movie in a private house in the south of France. We all sat around with our drinks after dinner and at the end of the film it was a great strain to remember our manners enough to say goodnight to our host before the rush for the stairs. When you've actually got something going then you can ask for what you like and answer his needs, but I think cold-blooded discussions of what you like in bed when you're not in the mood only create greater distance. You might discover you like dressing up, or that he does. There was a glorious moment at a party Maurice and I gave during *The Avengers* when Patrick Macnee was talking to probably the only 'proper' person there. Recognizing, no doubt, that she was shockable, he was wickedly informing her of the places where one could obtain a schoolgirl's or a nun's outfit or, as he so charmingly put it, 'Whatever you fancy, dear lady.' Her face was a picture.

Of course it's true to say that just as absence makes the heart grow fonder it also whets the appetite. Because I don't live with anyone and am very busy – as is my longstanding fella – our time together is particulary precious. Denial needn't be a disaster, unless of course you are being neglected by the person lying next to you. I was propositioned recently by someone I found quite attractive, but somebody new

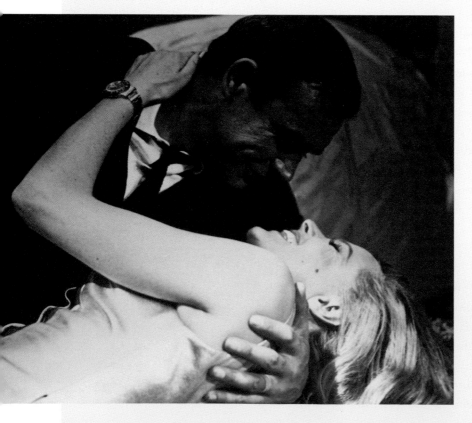

Talking of passion – Pussy Galore gets her teeth into James Bond!

would have to be an absolute knock-out before I dared to launch anew. The highest requirement on my list from any new person in my life would have to be a sense of humour. Indeed, that has always been the case.

There has only really been one departure from that in my life. One particular lover I had between and after marriages was wonderful, beautiful, with a smile you could die for and a body to match and the most delicious mouth I have ever known – I can still smell his skin. But if you let him he just talked and talked in a deadly serious fashion. You just had to occupy that mouth to stop him. Lust is a disaster when you are young, because it is frequently mistaken for love, lasting love. So often, after decisions have been made and unions forged, the physical attractions die away and there is no solid basis of shared interests or friendship.

Once when I was in Melbourne a journalist came to interview me. Despite the fact that he was dressed in shorts and long socks I thought we were having a very profound conversation about falling in love and sexual attraction. I was saying that it is such a pity that young people often confuse sexual attraction with love. The next day I went into a newsagent and saw a banner headline shouting 'HONOR LOVES LUST'. Well, yes, but only for openers!

I'm difficult to love, I think. A school report of mine once said that I was somewhat diffident and since I am also to a great extent a perfectionist it's a pretty rocky combination. I'm also cautious; over the years you can't help wondering if people are expecting you to be the characters you've played, but I'm not Pussy Galore, Cathy Gale or Laura West, thank heavens.

My home

The way we live our lives, our homes and our environments are all very important to us. I love to be surrounded by my books, family photographs and various mementoes from a full life. I live in a bright, airy apartment which is perfect for me. It's not so big that it takes me hours to clean, but it's more than adequate for my needs. My home is more than a base. Although I love to travel and discover new places it is terribly important. I always

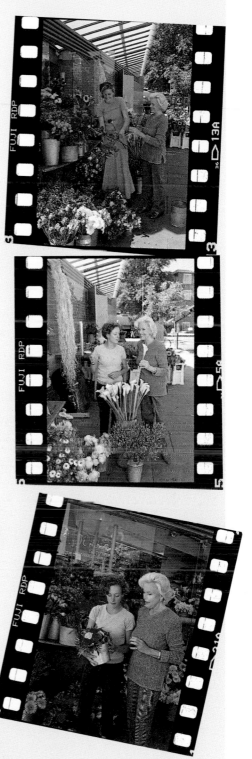

want to come back home and would never want to live anywhere else.

I suppose I could have a country cottage or a place abroad if I wanted, but I don't need more repairs to worry about. In any case, who wants to go back to the same spot all the time when there are so many beautiful places to see? These days I like to keep things as simple as possible. Why overcomplicate your life when you don't have to? I have so many friends who seem to spend the entire weekend doing jobs around the second home.

My home is a wonderful sanctuary where I can shut out the world and do anything I want. I am not overlooked, so I can walk about stark naked if I want to. It is decorated in soothing pale colours which I find terribly easy on the eye. A combination of soft yellow walls and pale blue sofas is very conducive to relaxation. I've always tried to live in soothing surroundings and don't care for brash things. I like continuity in design and for one colour to be used throughout, as I think it's very restful and gives the impression of space. I'm not keen on dark colours and couldn't bear to live somewhere gloomy like a dark basement. Light and sunshine affect my mood tremendously; maybe because I'm born under the sun sign of Leo I feel alive in the light and it has a very beneficial effect on my mood.

Entertainment at home

During evenings when I simply wish to relax I'll sometimes switch on the TV but I'm very selective about what I view. I never watch soap operas and only put on the TV if there is something particular I wish to see. I think it's so easy to slump down in front of the TV and watch everything that comes on, especially if you are tired. Before you know it the evening is over and you have achieved nothing. If I want a background to work to I'll play music, or when I'm doing the ironing I'll opt for the spoken word on the radio.

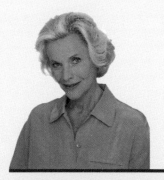

'I love to spend time at home. My home is my sanctuary and I'd never want to live anywhere else.'

One thing I love to watch on TV, however, is sport. I enjoy athletics, the track events in particular. It doesn't matter which distance I'm watching, although the 100 metres is very exciting. I've been a keen football fan for as long as I can remember. Maurice and I used to go to Fulham's Craven Cottage every Saturday and sometimes to away matches too, so I certainly know my 'off sides' from my 'goal kicks'. I don't follow their fortunes so much now but I love watching any really good football match. In Spain during Euro 96, we went to an English bar for the England v Spain match and I was heard to sing ''Ere we go, 'ere we go, 'ere we go' three times – although I must admit that the odd glass of wine had been taken! There's something very exciting about being with a mob who are willing the same team on. I also love tennis and quite enjoy motor racing – as my son is a Grand Prix fanatic he fills me in on everything. Events that seem monumentally boring at first become very exciting when you understand the problems, skills and nuances involved.

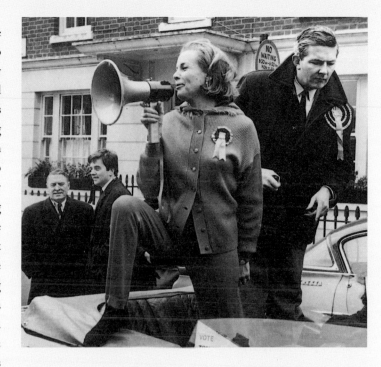

Doing my bit: here I am supporting my local Liberal candidate before the 1964 election.

Maybe it's a follow on from my love of sport that I also enjoy the excitement of speed. It's very juvenile, I know, but I think it's because the only vehicle I had experience of as a child, apart from a bus, was my Uncle Dick's motorbike. He visited us rarely, but it was so thrilling when he did. He had wonderfully dark wavy hair and a voice so low it purred, and he would take us out in his side car. I still remember the sensation of the wind in my face and the sound of that engine with a thrill. It's probably why I volunteered to be a dispatch rider in the war when I was 17. God knows what would have happened to the country if they had to rely on me. I used to put my feet up on the petrol tank and roar down Western Avenue. In training they had called me 'Top Gear Tessie'. Luckily there was a lot less traffic on the roads then.

Those first bikes belonged to the Home Office and we used to deliver blood, not important documents. Later I had a Honda and sometimes used to take the kids for a ride, though I'm not sure how much they enjoyed it – children like to conform and they didn't know any other mum who did that. Besides, as passengers they didn't get much of a view. I gave up riding a motorbike when it became too heavy for me. It's no fun lying in the road with a bike on top of you if you are unable to get out from under it.

In 1965 I remember being asked to drive a convertible Mercedes by the *Evening Standard* the day before the 70mph limit was imposed. They sent a photographer along, coincidentally called Peter Blackman, who snapped me as I zoomed up and down the M4 for hours at top speed – quite a treat.

Another time, when I was learning to fly, I was having such a wonderful time taxiing along the runway that as the trees and hedges ahead of us came rushing into view the instructor was finally forced to call over my shoulder 'Have you thought of taking off, Miss Blackman?' Even today I own a powerful car (obviously I don't speed) and I love to drive.

Money

I love having money – who doesn't? I'm particularly fond of a quote by the singer Sophie Tucker which goes 'From birth to age 18, a girl needs good parents. From 18 to 35 she needs good looks. From 35 to 55 she needs a good personality and from 55 on she needs good cash'. I have to account for every penny I spend, apart from little bits of cash, because of tax and VAT and I know exactly where all my investments are. If your mind blurs as mine does the moment percentages or any financial matters are discussed you have to find some dear, patient soul in the investment business who will take time to explain things to you as if to a child – and then you should get a second opinion, perhaps from a clued-up friend or acquaintance. My stockbroker knows not to advise me to buy shares in arms, tobacco and such-like. My decisions upset him sometimes, but I

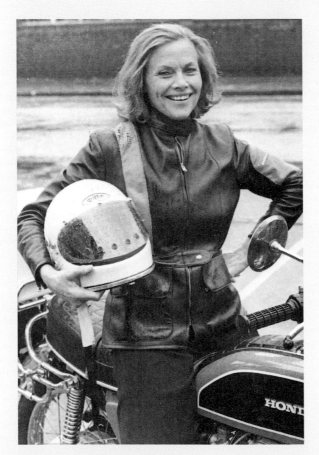

'Top Gear Tessie' ready for action!

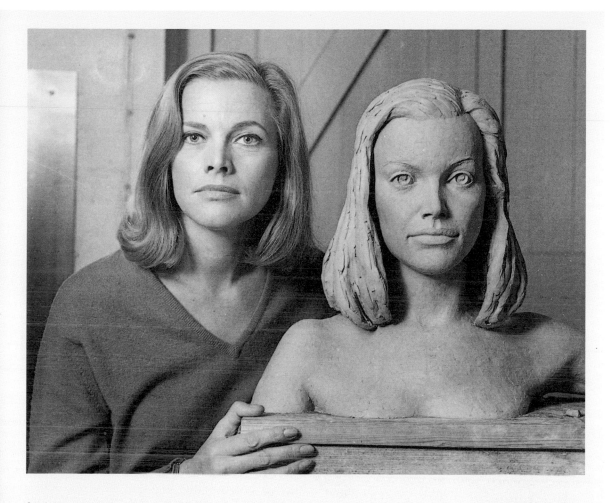

think he's lovely and amazingly tolerant of my ignorance on most financial matters.

This beautiful sculpture was created by Richard Browne in 1963.

KNOWING MYSELF

Confidence

My level of confidence varies according to the particular situation I'm in, just the same as everyone else's does. If I'm meeting someone new and important or embarking upon a new role I can be distinctly apprehensive. From the point of view of knowing my job I am confident because I will always have worked at the role. It's self-defence, really. What actor wants to look a fool in front of hundreds of people? I couldn't bear to take on a new role without doing thorough preparation; it would make me feel very

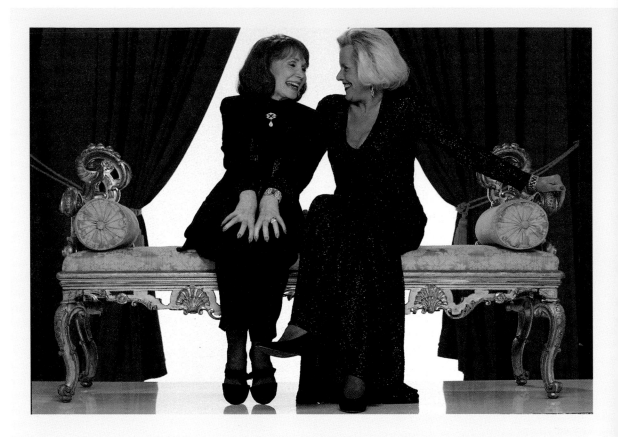

In the USA *The Upper Hand* was called *Who's The Boss?* and Katherine Helmond played the Laura West character.

ashamed of myself. Quite a lot of people manage to wing it a bit, but I can't – I have to know exactly what I'm doing. The key to success is hard work. It's an awful cliché which irritates us when people say it, but it is true, and it applies to every aspect of our lives.

That's not to say, however, that I can't be inspired to ad lib when I'm on stage. It is not advisable in a company to have such inspirations – you may throw the other actors and not be very popular! However, during my one-woman show I sometimes do something completely off the cuff that works well. But I like to have worked, to be prepared.

Coping

At this stage in life I suppose I could compare myself to an experienced athlete. They know what they have achieved in a race and, barring some hideous accident, know what they can produce. My situation is rather similar since I've worked so hard all my life. It doesn't matter how nervous

I feel about doing something new, I just have to think of all the things I've done which have been more difficult to give myself confidence.

When I got the part of Cathy Gale in *The Avengers* I replaced a man, Ian Hendry, who was very good. In those days, a woman never replaced a man in a part. It was felt that a female character would not pack the equivalent punch of a male character, and when I landed Cathy Gale it broke the mould. But I got that role during one of the most traumatic times of my life. The producer must have thought I had the quality required. Perhaps desperation had lent me a certain determination and assertiveness.

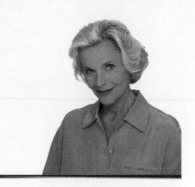

'I stand no nonsense from anyone: if I feel that I'm being taken advantage of the balloon goes up!'

My very first audition was memorable and very funny. Each actor was expected to play a scene of three minutes' duration. I did a scene from Maxwell Anderson's *Winter Set* and the director said afterwards, 'You were quite something. I knew you would be all right. You swept on with great confidence, demanded that we imagine the bridge here and gunfire there and then proceeded to do seven minutes against all the rules.'

I love my work even if I feel like hell before the curtain goes up or the director calls 'action' – once I'm on, I really enjoy it. Audiences are so warm – they have come to the event specifically to have a good time, after all. In comedy, when the first laugh comes it gives you a terrific charge – it's like being on a horse which suddenly goes from trotting to canter and if you are lucky you can progress to a gallop!

Positive thinking

I think that self-respect is as much about liking yourself and doing what you think is right as it is about how you allow others to treat you. There's no doubt that some people are natural victims, allowing others to push them around. I'm quite malleable provided I can find myself in agreement with what I'm asked to do, but I find it almost impossible to take direction which I can't feel is honest to the character. In everyday life I like to be accommodating, but if I feel that I'm being manipulated or taken advantage of the balloon goes up! That's

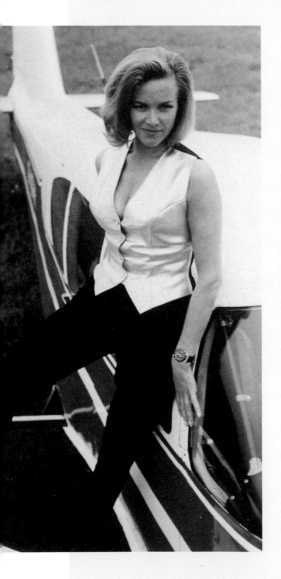

Pussy Galore: I've always enjoyed playing strong characters.

not always been the case; there have been times in my life when I've been in relationships that have gone wrong. I've cared very much about the other person and I've tried to change my personality and views in order to please him – but it never works. The consequence is that you make yourself miserable by losing track of who you are. When this has happened to me, I've invariably woken up one morning and thought, 'This is not ME. What is happening to ME?', kicked the appropriate person in the shins and promptly cut adrift.

In everyday life it is true that I can be quite determined and one-track-minded. I'm extremely conscious of fair play and justice and I can't stand bullies. I can recall leaping out of my car and sloshing a big boy who was mangling a small one. Not a good example for the boy – violence in response to violence – but I was enraged. Charm can oil all sorts of situations and though it's dangerously close to sexism there is no harm in using a spot of charm on a policeman or traffic warden or whoever. He may have had a bad day or has a sick child or his feet may be killing him – or he may just be a fan and one can't afford to alienate them!

Take control

There is a song that goes 'You've got to accentuate the positive.' I agree absolutely. Cancel 'I couldn't', 'I wouldn't' and 'I don't' from your vocabulary. A positive stance not only makes a better impression on everyone else but they in turn are affected by your attitude. Your dealings with them become more pleasant and satisfying, and this applies to both work and personal relationships.

Walk down the street – as my father used to say – as if you own it; shoulders back, head up, arms swinging. Don't scuttle about all hunched up with a worried frown.

The actress Dame Edith Evans played many characters who are said to be beautiful. She wasn't, but when she was on stage you believed she was because she believed it. It is essential that we like ourselves and if you determine to organize your life so that you are fit and healthy, well-groomed and presentable, and you adopt a positive attitude towards anything that life throws up, you will like yourself and be proud of your achievements.

We can all understand a soldier's pride when his buttons, badges, belt, boots and bearing are all immaculate. He knows that his appearance is important – if he doesn't, his sergeant major will soon tell him. Well, be your own sergeant major, your own critic, take control of your life and enjoy being in charge, as I do.

The future

There is so much that I still hope to do, from work to travelling, that it's driving me potty worrying whether I'll have the time. I am always looking for a new challenge. I've done theatre, musicals, TV, a one-person show, radio, commentary, commercials and voice-overs and I'm hoping to find something new. I'd love to try some more serious theatre work. Unfortunately there are very few Shakespearean roles for the older woman. A woman *can* play a male role – it rarely happens, but you never know, I might be rather good! I'd like to do something very different – I like to be surprised. I'm not frightened about taking chances; before I did *The Upper Hand* I wasn't known for doing comedy, but when I was sent the scripts they made me laugh. I deliberated because Laura West wasn't the main character but I haven't been bored at all. It's worked wonderfully well and as I do my show alongside I have the best of both worlds.

When I was young it was drummed into me not to waste time – so much so that I had a guilt complex if I sat and read something pleasurable instead of doing something useful. These days I've learnt to quieten that part of my conscience and realize that it's important to relax. It means that I can make the most of my days and fit in all the things that I want to do. I hope never to be one of those people who say 'I never did get to see the Niagara Falls' or whatever their dearest wish was. I intend to do so much more with my life.

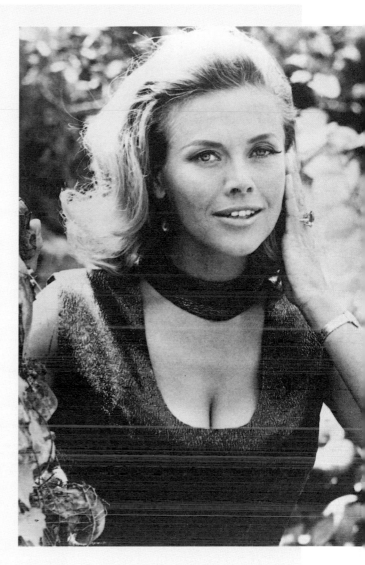

I've learnt not to fret about the future. I'm excited about tomorrow but I know that enjoying today is just as important.

ACKNOWLEDGEMENTS

The Publishers would like to thank everyone involved with the creation of the book.
Jimmie Dark (Wardrobe), Jeanette Stamp and Pat Postle (Make-Up), Claire Usher at MaxMara, John Rogers, Elaine Ingram, Alex Brunner, John Herron at UDC, Hill & Knowlton, Jane O'Gorman, Ian R Davey, Dr Frank Ryan and all at Carlton for their help.

PICTURE CREDITS